Keto Vegan Cookbook

Easy And Delicious Low Carb Keto Vegan Recipes

With 30 Days Meal Plan For Weight Loss

Table of Contents

Chapter 6 - Snacks and Desserts Vegan Keto Recipes 110

Introduction

I want to thank you and congratulate you for downloading the book, Keto Vegan Cookbook: Easy and Delicious Low Carb Keto Vegan Recipes With 30 Days Meal Plan For Weight Loss

When you have decided to cut out the use of animal products in your diet and go full vegan, it means that you will only eat food that are allowed in the keto-vegan diet. Although the ketogenic diet is mostly meat, going vegan would mean that you're going to put down food from animals, including dairy products and eggs.

Many people think that the vegan keto diet is difficult to follow and is highly restrictive. However, with proper planning and the right knowledge, you can turn it into a sustainable lifestyle.

This cookbook shows easy vegan-keto meals that are easy to prepare. Here, you will find 25 recipes for breakfast, lunch, snacks/desserts, and dinner. Get started right now and prepare your own vegan-keto meals with the help of this cookbook.

CHAPTER 1

Keto Vegan Basics

List of Food to Avoid – Vegan No-Nos

Trying to figure out what ingredients contain animal products can be a nightmare. This list of animal-product ingredients will help you on your journey to becoming a full-fledged vegan.

1. **Red Meat**

   Deer or venison meat

   - o Cattle/Cows - Beef lard, Beef cuts and veal.
   - o Charcuterie dried/smoked beef, and cold cuts. Examples include: corned beef, bacon, sausages, liver pate, and pastrami.
   - o Dairy products such as butter, cream, cheese, milk, and yogurt.

   Pigs (Farm or wild)

   - o Pork cuts including blood, liver, etc.
   - o Cold cuts, dried/smoked pork such as ham, salami, sausages, bacon, bologna, etc.

   Goat

   - o including goat cheese and milk

   Lamb and sheep

   - o including milk and cheese

Exotic animals

- such as those from alligator/crocodile, bear, bison, camel, frog, guinea pigs, horse, moose, snail, turtle, water buffalo, zebra, etc.

2. **White Meat**

Poultry, domesticated and wild

- Chicken eggs and Chicken meat including liver, gizzard, etc.
- Duck eggs, duck meat, duck fat and liver
- Turkey meat, ham and sausages
- Quail eggs and meat
- Birds' meat from goose, guinea fowl, ostrich, pigeon, etc.

Seafood

- Fish of all kinds
- Sea mammals such as seals, dolphins, polar bears, walruses, whales, etc.
- Crustaceans such as crab, crawfish, crayfish, krill, lobster, prawn, shrimp, etc.
- Fish roe such as caviar and roe from grouper, lumpfish, salmon, tuna, capelin, etc.
- Echinoderm such as sea urchin and sea cucumber
- Shellfish such as octopus, squid, mussels, scallops, clams, oysters, sea snails, etc.

o Seafood-based products such as canned and/or pickled fish, bottled,
brined, fish chowder, dried seafood, fish broths/soups, fish sauce, and
shrimp paste, etc.

3. Insects, and insect by-products

The following are food items containing amounts of animal/insects by
products:

o Beer and wine. Some beer manufacturers use casein from cow's milk,
industrial food grade gelatin, and albumen from egg whites.

o Bread and baked goodies that are commercially-produced. This
includes those that are frozen, cake mixes, and microwave-ready
bread.

o Artificially colored food and drinks specifically those that are in red
shades such as ruby red, pink, deep violet, etc. This food additive is
known in names such as crimson ink, crimson lake, carmine, carmine
red, E120, cochineal, natural red 4, and C.I. 75470 among others.
Although considered safe to be consumed by humans, vegans would
not find this pleasant.

o Candies, cakes, chocolate drinks, energy drinks, and granola bars are
just few of the many products containing this food additive that come
from a cochineal bug.

o Frozen fruits and vegetables are likewise treated with this to make
them look more appealing when sold on the market.

- Commercial candies, gelatin, and gummy bears also contain collagen extracted from animal skins, bones, and ligaments and are usually a byproduct of cattle. Collagen is a kind of protein that makes sweets look glossy, gelatins to wiggle, and candies to stretch.
- Even salad dressings have traces of animals such as crab, fish sauce, and other powdered forms.
- Honey-flavored food and drinks. Honey is used in many products tagged as healthy, but they are a no-no to vegan people.
- Junk food like chips, although typically unhealthy, contain food additives and an insect-based food coloring called casein. So although other chips are labeled as vegan or vegan-safe, they are still not worth it. As vegan, it is advised that you do away with chips, popcorns, French fries and even beverages with flavorings. Or, better yet, avoid fast food meals altogether.
- Commercially manufactured nuts flavored with honey, cheese, and barbecue also contain gelatin to make them look shiny. Buy raw nuts instead or if you wanted the roasted version, roast them at home.

List of Food Items That Should Be in Your Pantry

- o Canned/bottled beans, fruits, and vegetables. These will make your life easier especially if you do not have the luxury of time to soak and cook beans for hours. Always rinse and drain canned vegetables before using. If you are going to buy canned fruits, buy those in light syrup.

- o Condiments such as kimchi, mustard, horseradish, miso paste, and sauerkraut are all vegan-safe.

- o Fresh produce. This typically includes fruits, vegetables, herbs, and beans.

- o Dried pulses and grains such as lentils, dried beans, nuts, and seeds among others.

- o Dark colored grains such as red, brown, or wild rice. Black and red quinoa also count.

- o Frozen produce such as fruits, vegetables, and peas. However, too much freezing could compromise the nutritional value and taste of the food. So use frozen produce sparingly.

- o Nut cheeses, nut butter, or soy-based margarine, almond milk, cashew milk, flax milk, coconut milk, hemp milk, hazelnut milk, oat milk, macadamia nut milk, rice milk, soy milk quinoa milk, and.

- o Light-colored oats and couscous. Avoid using instant ones.

- o Egg-free multi-grained pasta. Pasta dishes are part and parcel of the vegan diet. They are versatile and are easy to cook.

- Dried, fresh or canned/bottled mushrooms. They are a good source of protein and fiber. They also make wonderful ingredients to almost all recipes.
- Raw nuts and seeds. Just make sure you do the roasting at home with homemade nut butters and cheeses.

- Soy products such as soy cheese, soy sauce, edamame, soy milk, soy nuts, tofu, and tempeh among others.
- Organic flavoring such as sun-dried tomatoes, kosher salt, pesto sauce, tomato sauce/paste, and miso paste.
- Sweeteners such as date syrup, green *stevia*, palm sugar, raw cane sugar syrup, and bacon syrup.
- Cooked or processed sweeteners such as pure maple syrup, agave syrup, coconut sugar, barley malt syrup, brown rice syrup, blackstrap molasses, molasses, unwashed/unrefined cane sugar, and unwashed/unrefined palm sugar are recommended.

CHAPTER 2

The Basics and Benefits of

Low Carb Keto Meal Prepping

The Ketogenic Diet, or Keto, is fast becoming the alternative diet for many people. It has helped many lose weight, overcome PCOS (polycystic ovarian syndrome), enhance their athletic performance, and manage Alzheimer's disease and other neurological conditions.

If you are someone who is currently on the Keto diet, then you would understand how difficult it can be to maintain, especially since we are often surrounded by high carb food. Keto dieters more often than not would need to prepare their own meals at home to ensure their enjoyment of delicious, healthy, low carb and high fat food.

The good news, however, is that you can choose to **meal prep** your low carb keto meals. That way, can save a lot of money, time, and effort as you continue to be on the keto diet. Meal prepping is a practical way to prepare food at home because it enables you to cook large batches for only a few times per week (sometimes even once a week) and then store individual portions of the food properly in the refrigerator or freezer. Then, throughout the week, all you will have to do is reheat those servings and enjoy them. Best of all, some foods, such as salads and snacks, do not even need reheating at all.

How to Meal Prep the Right Way

Some people have quit meal prepping simply because they do not follow a practical and efficient process. You can avoid becoming one of them by creating one, and these guidelines can help you do so.

1: Choose where and when to do your weekly grocery shopping

Where would you like to buy your ingredients? Take note of the closest markets in your area that offer the best quality your food budget can afford. Then, determine the best day and time to purchase all the ingredients you need there. For instance, if your free day is on a Saturday morning and you know not a lot of people do their grocery shopping at 10 a.m. in that market, then you can schedule your weekly trips then.

2: Create a grocery list template.

Whether it is on your phone or a physical list, you should have a template on which to list down the ingredients you need for the recipes you will be meal prepping. Take note of the amount, generic names, and brands if you must. Then, sit down with your chosen recipes for the week and take note.

3: Shop in bulk.

Once you have a list of the ingredients you need, all you have to do is buy them during your chosen date and time. Then, store them appropriately in your kitchen pantry and refrigerator as soon as you get home.

4: Choose two Meal Prep Days.

Before you go grocery shopping, make sure you have already chosen your meal prep day for the week. Is it going to be on a Sunday afternoon? If so, then make sure you have bought the ingredients a day before. That way, you will not be so exhausted by the time you start cooking.

5: Prepare your individual food containers.

You will make your own life so much easier if you divide your meal prepped meals into individual containers because you will then be able to do a "grab and go" system throughout the week. Choose guaranteed food-safe, airtight containers suitable for the types of foods you want to enjoy. Also, label the containers so you would not end up storing your delicate muffins in one that smells strongly of garlic and pepper.

There you have it: meal prepping made easy. If you are not the only one who will enjoy these meal prepped meals, then you can definitely work together with whoever you are sharing them with. That way, you can cut on cost and time so much more effectively.

Common Mistakes in Meal Prepping

There are definitely safety measures to take when meal prepping. After all, you are dealing with something that you put into your body. So, here are some common mistakes you must avoid while meal prepping your low carb Keto meals.

Mistake 1: Storing cooked food for more than 4 days in the fridge.

The safest maximum number of days for storing most cooked food in the refrigerator (40 degrees F or lower) is 4 days. The food should also be stored in an airtight container to significantly slow down oxidation. Any longer than 4 days and you might risk food poisoning.

Mistake 2: Reheating food more than once

Cooked food should never be reheated more than once. Otherwise, you could risk not just losing the nutritional value and flavor but also the chance of food poisoning. You should also reheat the food until the internal temperature reaches 165 degrees F to ensure that it is completely thawed and safe to eat.

Mistake 3: Going to the grocery store without a detailed list

You could waste a lot of money and food when you overbuy certain ingredients. It is therefore critical for you to take note of the amount required for the meal prep before you step into the grocery store.

Mistake 4: Storing food improperly

Oxygen quickly breaks down the food and causes bacteria to flourish, that is why you must minimize the food's exposure to oxygen as soon as it is cool enough to be stored. This can be achieved by using airtight containers and freezer bags. You can also do the water immersion technique to make bagged food airtight before sealing. Check any online video on how to do this.

Mistake 5: Failing to add variety

It is important to eat different food within the week for two reasons. First is, you could easily grow bored with the same meals every day. Second is, you will not be able to give your body a variety of nutrients if you eat the same types of food daily. So, do not hesitate to try other recipes. Better yet, always include a fresh salad with most of your meals so you will not only add variety to flavor, but also to nutrients.

At this point, you must be ready to start low carb Keto meal prepping. So, without further ado, go ahead and get started!

CHAPTER 3

Vegan Keto Breakfast Recipes

Chia Blueberry Pudding

Ingredients:

- 6 oz plain soy yogurt
- 6 oz frozen blueberries
- 3 oz fresh blueberries
- 2 Tbsp. white chia seeds
- 2 Tbsp. pure maple syrup
- ¼ tsp pure vanilla extract

Directions:

1. Blend the frozen blueberries in a food processor until smooth.
2. Add the yogurt and maple syrup, then blend until smooth.
3. Stir in the chia seeds and vanilla extract, then spoon into mason jars. Top with fresh blueberries, then refrigerate overnight. Serve the next morning.

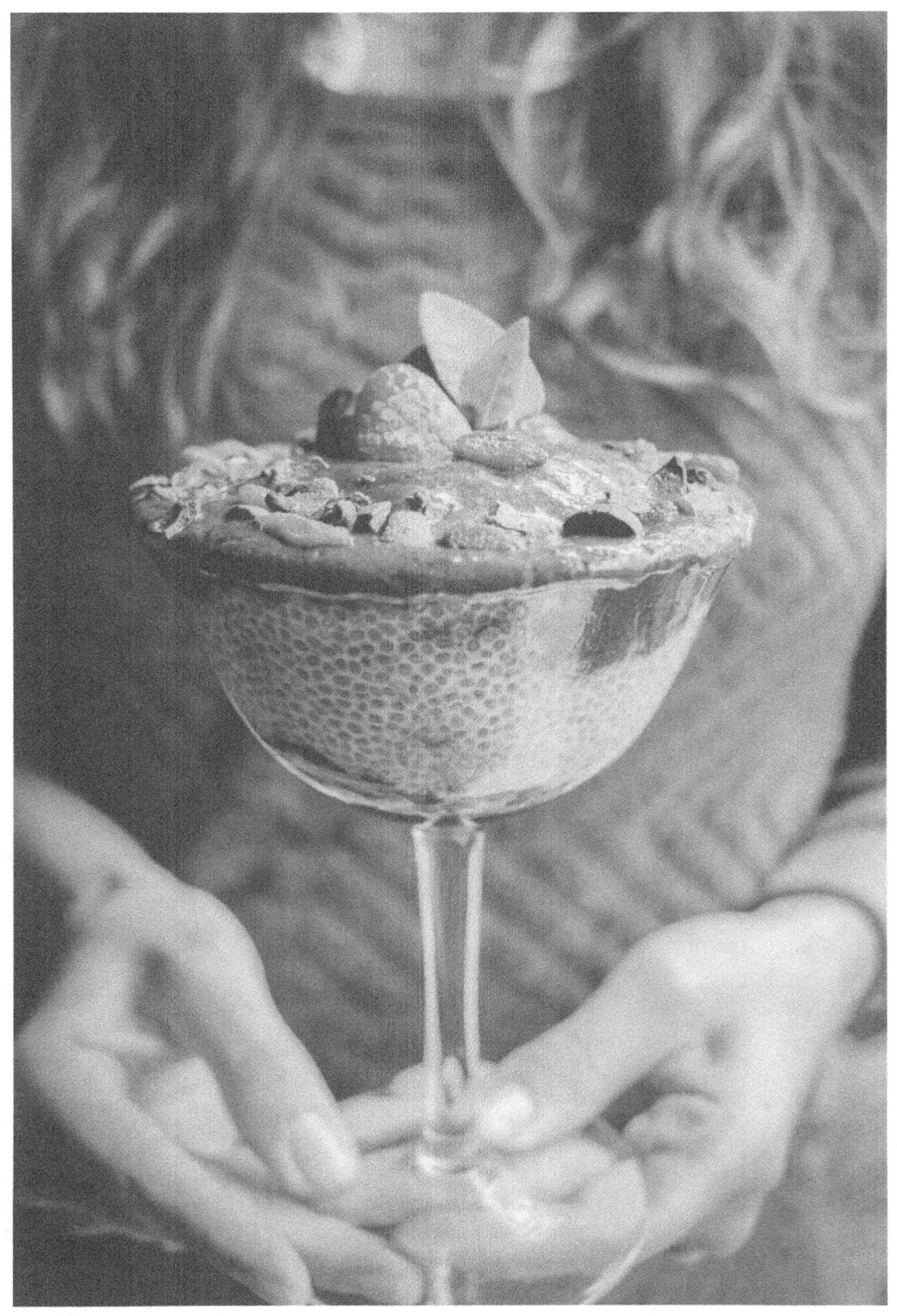

Plantain Flapjacks

Ingredients:

- 1 overripe plantain
- ½ cup applesauce (substitute for eggs)
- 1 Tbsp. coconut butter
- 1 Tbsp. coconut flour
- 1 Tbsp. canned coconut milk
- 3/4 Tbsp. cinnamon
- 1/4 tsp baking soda
- 1/4 tsp baking powder
- Pinch of salt
- 1 1/2 Tbsp. coconut oil

For the syrup

- 1/4 plantain, diced
- 1 Tbsp. maple syrup
- 1 tsp cinnamon

Directions:

1. Place skillet over medium heat and add coconut oil.

2. Meanwhile, cut ends of the plantain and peel. Slice into three equal pieces and put the pieces in the hot skillet.

3. Sprinkle with a bit of salt and cinnamon. Cook for 2 minutes, flip and sprinkle some more cinnamon and salt, and cook the other side for 2 more minutes.

4. Take plantain off pan and place on a plate. Set aside to cool, then place 2 pieces in a bowl.

5. Mash the two pieces and add the applesauce, coconut milk, coconut flour, baking soda, cinnamon, baking powder, and butter. Add a pinch of salt and mix well to create a paste.

6. Reheat skillet over medium flame and add a bit of coconut oil. Spoon some of the pancake batter on top and cook until bubbles form.

7. Flip and cook for 1 minute then transfer onto a plate. Repeat until all pancakes are cooked. Set aside to cool for a bit before you store in a microwavable container.

8. Dice the remaining plantain piece and combine it with the cinnamon and maple syrup. Stir and put in a covered container.

9. Refrigerate the pancakes and syrup. Before serving, spoon syrup on top and reheat in the microwave.

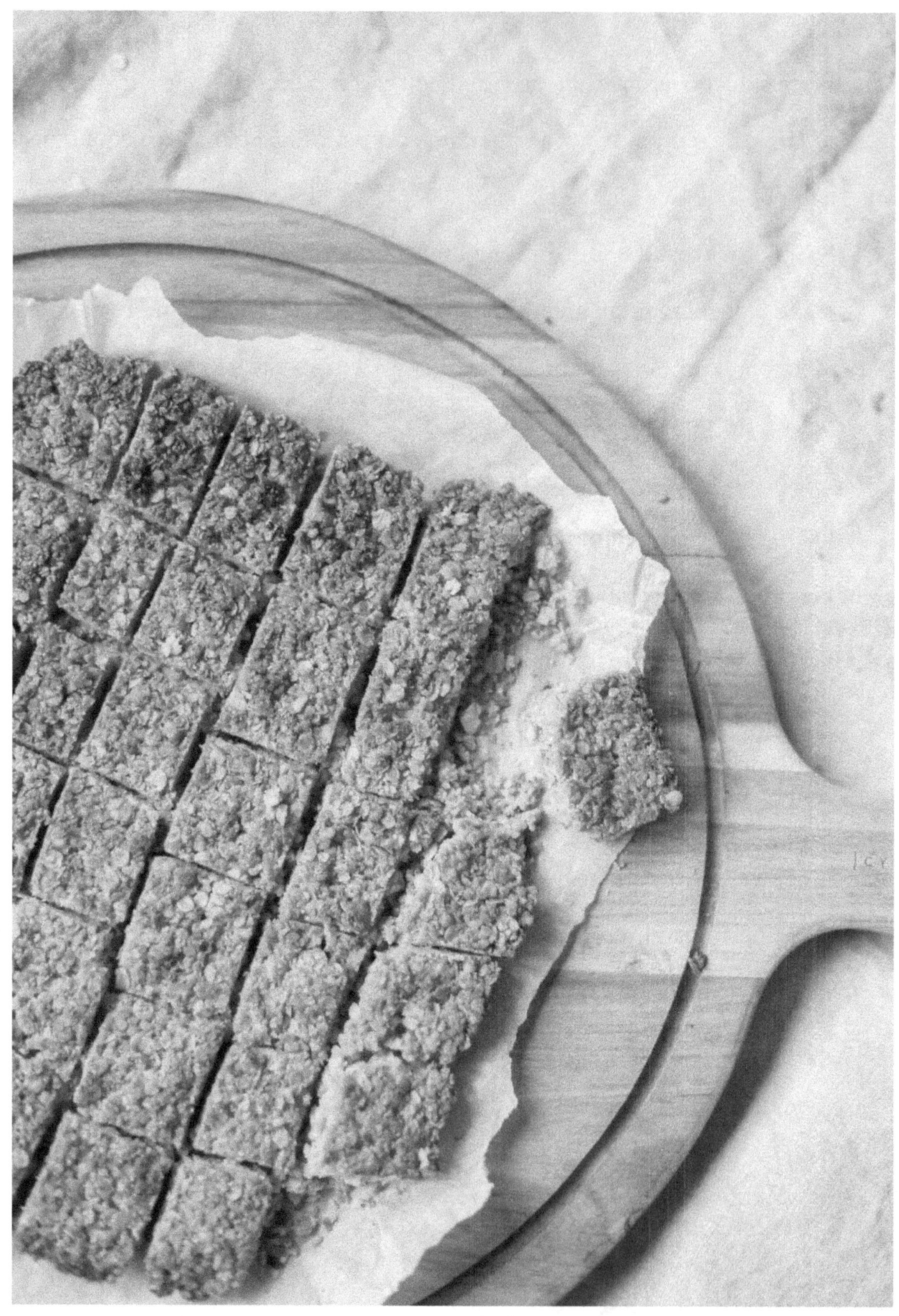

Baby Spinach and Watercress Salad with Black Currant Vinaigrette

Ingredients:

Vinaigrette

- 2 garlic, grated
- ⅛ cup packed fresh cilantro, minced
- 2 tablespoons black currant vinegar
- ½ teaspoon red pepper flakes
- ¼ cup lemon juice, fresh squeezed
- Pinch of sea salt
- Pinch of black pepper
- ⅛ cup extra virgin olive oil

Salad

- 2 pounds watercress, shredded
- 3 sprigs, flat-leaf parsley, leaves and tender stems only, torn
- 1 head baby spinach leaves

Directions:

1. Pour dressing ingredients into small bottle with tight fitting lid. Seal and shake bottle until salt and sugar dissolves.
2. Place remaining ingredients into salad bowl; drizzle in dressing. Toss to combine. Place equal portions into bowls. Serve immediately.

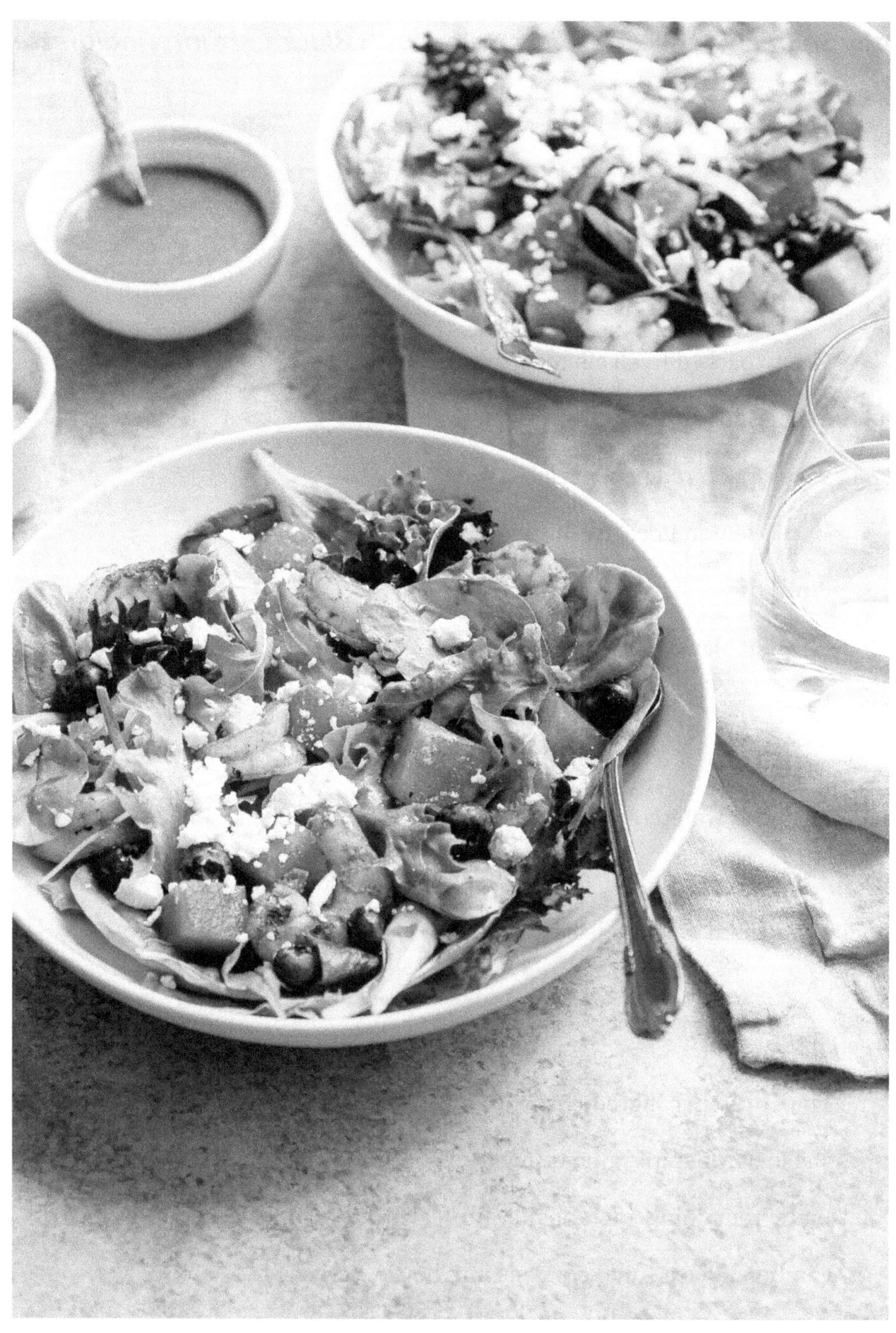

Breakfast Avocado and Tomato Salad

Ingredients:

- ½ avocado, minced

- 2 sprigs cilantro, minced

- 2 tablespoons lemon juice, fresh squeezed

- 1 leek, minced

- 1 ripe tomato, deseeded, minced

- 1 Serrano chili, deseeded, minced

- Pinch of sea salt

- Pinch of white pepper

Directions:

1. Mix avocado salad ingredients in a small bowl, mashing some (not all) avocado as you go. Taste; adjust seasoning if needed.

2. Spread equal portions on grain-free bread slices of choice or eat as salad mix. Serve.

Creamy Broccoli Soup

Ingredients:

- 3 cups broccoli florets, chopped
- 1 onion, minced
- 1 Tbsp. coconut flour
- ½ cup unsweetened soymilk
- 2 cups vegetable broth, low sodium
- Sea salt
- 1 Tbsp. coconut oil

Directions:

1. Combine the onion, broccoli, and vegetable broth in a stockpot and cover tightly. Place over high flame and bring to a boil.
2. Once boiling, reduce to medium low flame and simmer for 30 minutes, or until the vegetables are extra tender.
3. Meanwhile, place a saucepan over low flame and add the coconut oil. Stir in the flour and mix well. Pour in the soymilk and stir until smooth. Set aside.
4. Once the vegetables are cooked, turn off the heat and allow to cool slightly. Once cooked, puree the solids in a food processor, blender or by using an immersion blender.
5. Reheat the soup over low flame, pour in the soymilk mixture. Season to taste with salt, then serve right away.

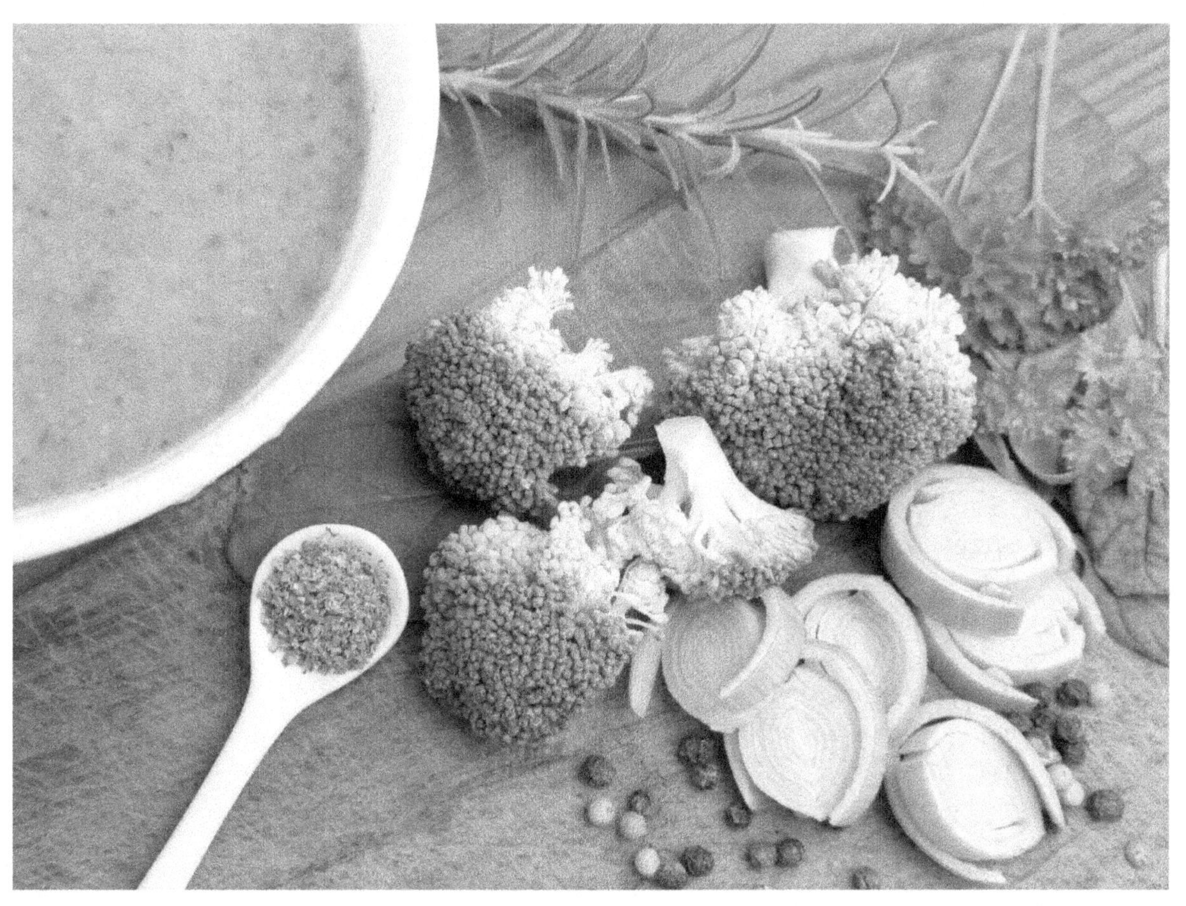

Veggie Tofu Scramble

Ingredients:

- ½ Tbsp. olive oil
- 2 cups firm tofu, drained
- 1 onion, minced
- 1 tomato, diced
- ¼ cup diced zucchini
- ¼ cup diced red bell pepper
- ½ Tbsp. nutritional yeast
- ¼ tsp turmeric
- ¼ tsp cumin
- Sea salt
- ground black pepper

Directions:

1. Heat the olive oil in a cast iron skillet over medium flame, then sauté the vegetables until tender.
2. Add the spices and nutritional yeast and mix well. Add the tofu and scramble well, mixing with the vegetables. Season to taste with salt and pepper, then serve.

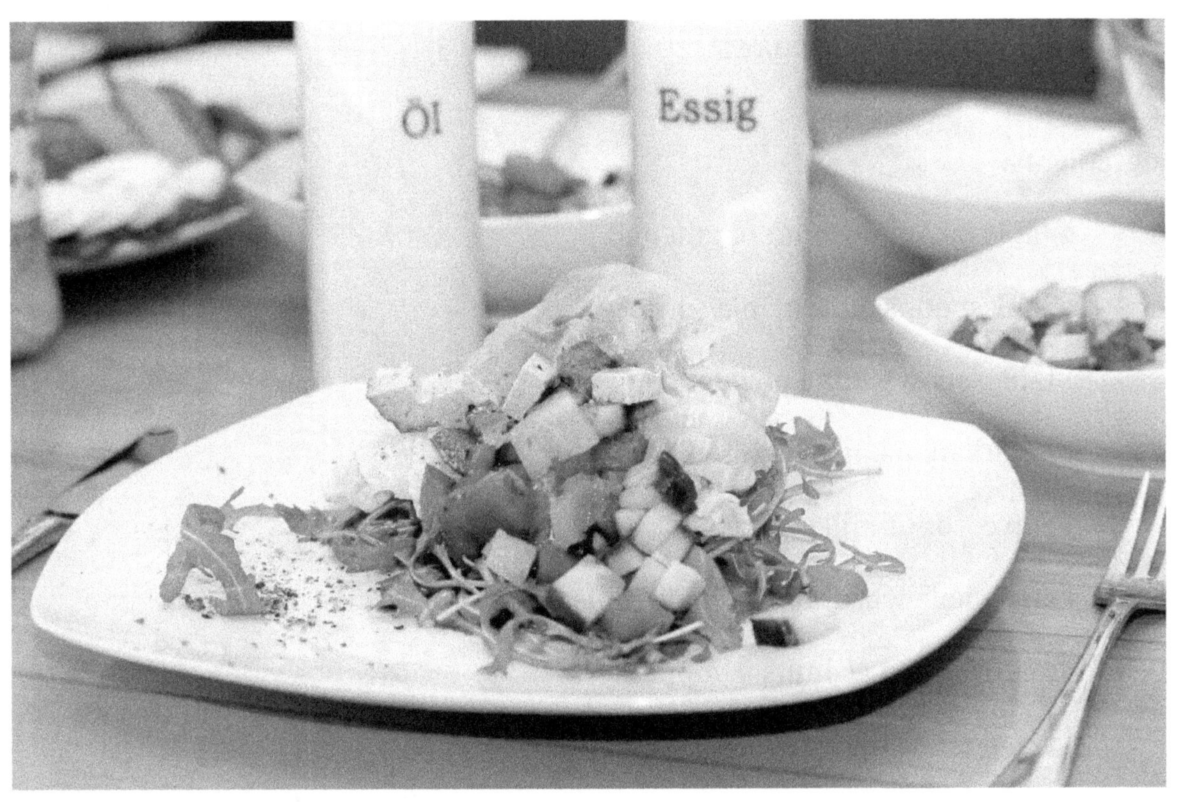

Öl
Essig

Banana-Walnuts Pancakes

Ingredients:

- 2 tablespoons coconut oil, melted
- 2 tablespoons pure maple syrup
- 1 tablespoon baking powder
- 1 large banana, mashed well
- 1 cup coconut milk
- 1 cup whole wheat flour, finely milled
- ½ cup toasted walnuts, chopped
- 1 teaspoon vanilla extract
- ¼ teaspoon kosher salt

Directions:

1. Combine ingredients in large mixing bowl. Do not over mix. Lightly grease skillet with oil and set over medium heat.
2. Divide batter into 6 equal portions, about ¼ cup each. Pour into hot skillet. Flip when edges are set, and center is no longer runny. Do not press down on pancakes.
3. Plate. Drizzle desired amount of pure maple syrup. Serve.

Scrambled Eggless Eggs

Ingredients:

- 2 tablespoons olive oil
- 2 garlic cloves, minced
- ½ medium onion, chopped
- 1 package tofu, crumbled
- ½ teaspoon turmeric
- 1/8 teaspoon cumin
- 2 tablespoons Braggs

Directions:

1. In a large sauce pan, heat the oil.
2. Saute garlic and onions for 3 minutes or until translucent and fragrant.
3. Add tofu, turmeric, cumin, and Braggs. Saute for 5 minutes or until tofu is lightly seared. Continue stirring for 5 minutes or until the liquid has evaporated. Serve.

Cranberry and Blueberry Pancakes

Ingredients:

- 2 tablespoons coconut oil, melted

- 2 tablespoons palm sugar, crumbled

- 1 tablespoon baking powder

- 1 cup coconut milk

- 1 cup   whole wheat flour, finely milled

- ½ cup frozen blueberries, thawed

- ½ cup frozen cranberries, thawed

- 1 teaspoon vanilla extract

- ¼ teaspoon kosher salt

Directions:

1. Except for berries, combine ingredients in large mixing bowl. Do not over mix. Gently fold in blueberries and cranberries. Lightly grease skillet with oil and set over medium heat.

2. Divide batter into 6 equal portions, about ¼ cup each. Pour into hot skillet. Flip when edges are set, and center is no longer runny.

3. Do not press down on pancakes. Plate portions. Serve.

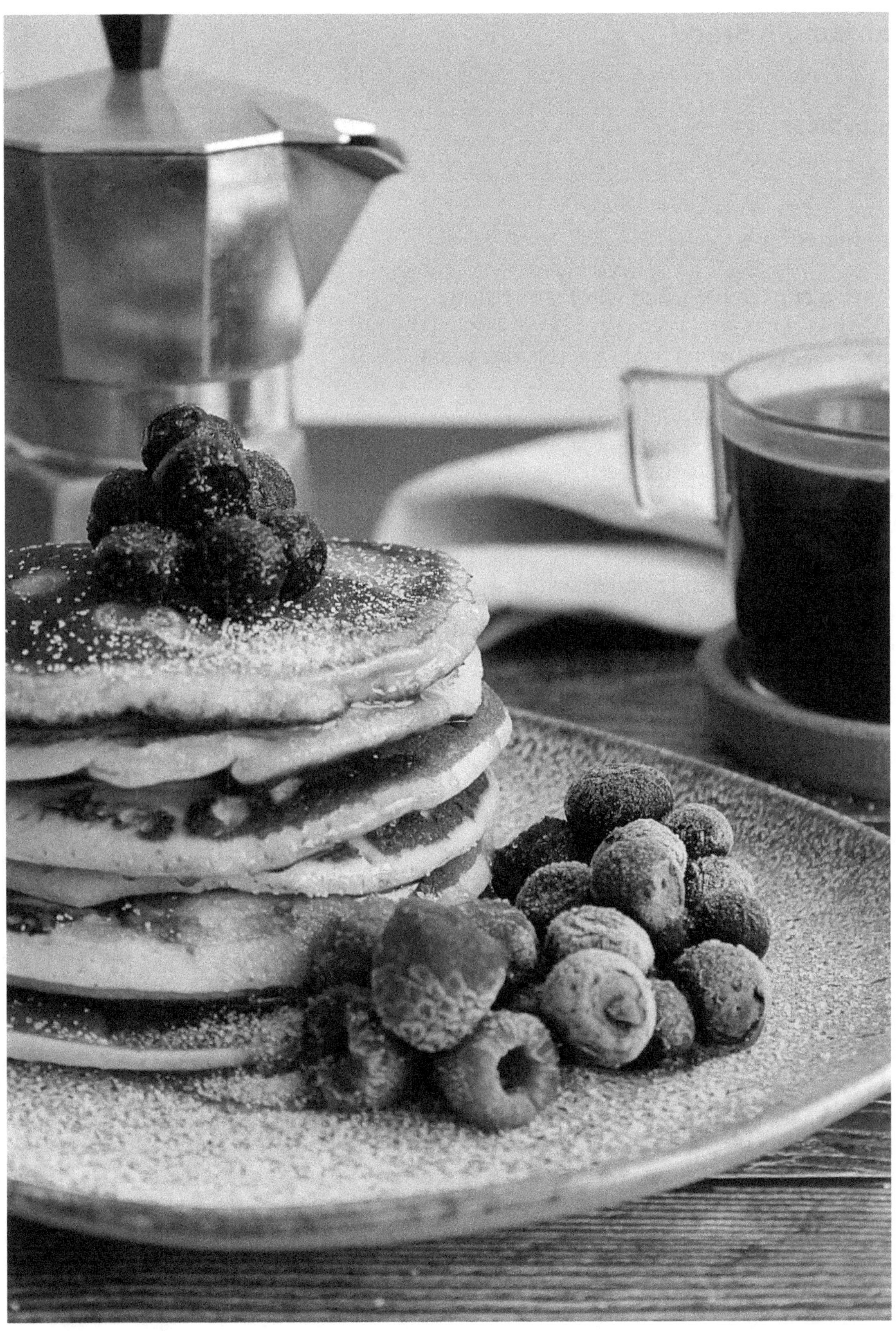

Cardamom Bread

Ingredients:

Dry ingredients

- 4 cups unbleached wholegrain flour
- 2¼ teaspoons packet active dry yeast
- 1½ teaspoon maple syrup
- 1 teaspoon kosher salt

Wet ingredients

- 1¾ cups freshly boiled water
- 2 tablespoons coconut oil, melted

Aromatics

- ⅛ teaspoon cardamom powder
- ⅛ teaspoon cinnamon powder
- dash of clove powder

Directions:

1. Combine dry ingredients into large mixing bowl. Make well in center. Pour in wet ingredients.

2. With a wooden spoon, gradually mix dry and wet ingredients until dough comes together. Turn out dough on floured surface; make depression in middle. Add in aromatics; knead until elastic, about 7 to 10 minutes Add flour if dough is too sticky.

3. Lightly grease (same) bowl with oil. Place dough in. Cover bowl with saran wrap. Let dough rise in a warm place for 1 to 1½ hours, or until double in size. Lightly grease bread loaf pans.

4. Punch dough down; turn out on floured surface. Divide in half. Form dough into rough loaf, stretching, and tucking in edges underneath; place in prepared loaf pans. Let dough rise for 20 minutes, covered loosely with saran wrap.

5. Preheat oven to 190°C / 375°F for 10 minutes. Place pans on middle rack of oven. Bake for 30 to 40 minutes, or until bread top is golden brown.

6. Remove pans from oven and set on cooling racks. When pan is cool enough to handle, remove loaves. Allow bread to cool further before slicing.

Raisin Rice Pudding

Ingredients:

- 3 cups soy milk

- 1 ½ teaspoons cinnamon

- 2 cups cooked brown rice

- 1 tablespoon vanilla extract

- 1 cup slivered almonds

- 1 cup raisins

- ¼ cup sweetener

Directions:

1. Add milk, cinnamon, brown rice, vanilla extract, almonds, raisins, and sweetener in a saucepan. Bring to a boil.

2. Reduce to a simmer for 15 minutes or until the pudding thickens. Stir occasionally. Cool for serving.

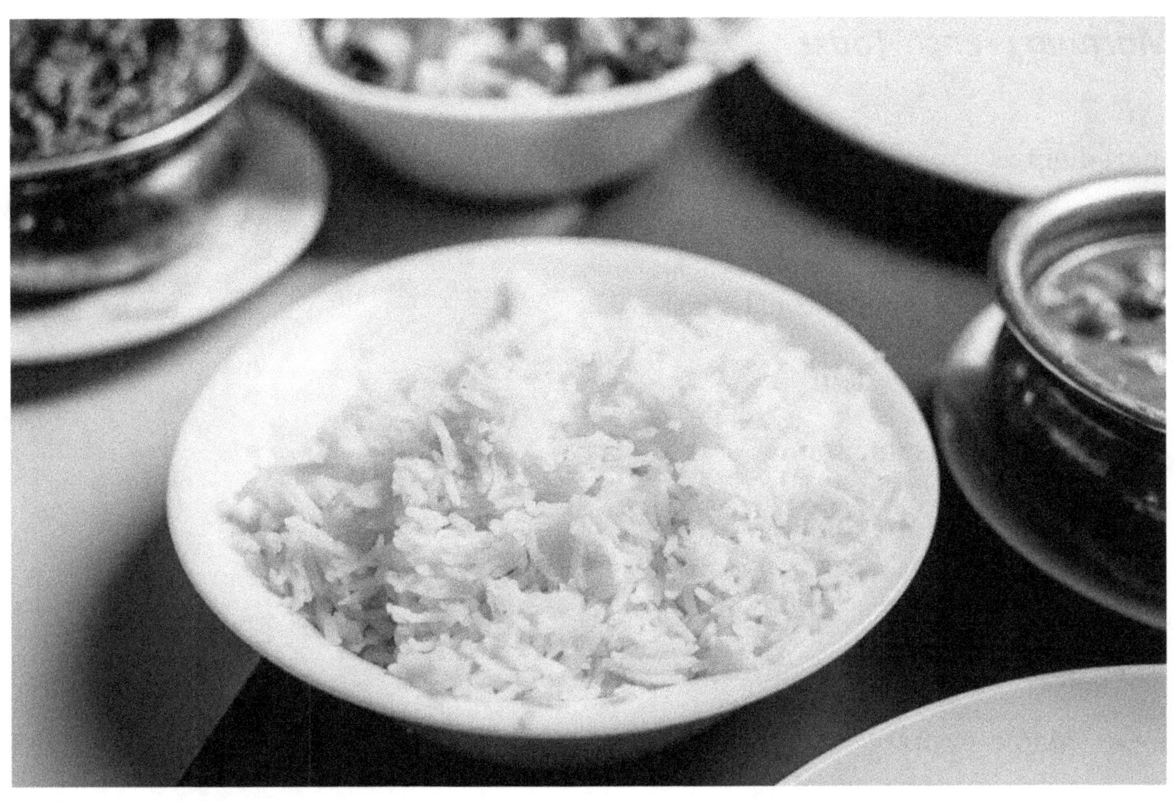

Morning French Toast

Ingredients:

- 1 ½ cups soy milk
- 1 tablespoon nutritional yeast
- 2 tablespoons flour
- 1 teaspoon cinnamon
- 1 teaspoon sweetener
- 5 bread slices
- Fruits of choice for garnish
- Maple syrup

Directions:

1. Combine soy milk, yeast, flour, and cinnamon in a bowl. Soak a slice of bread in batter.
2. Fry in a nonstick skillet until golden.
3. Flip and fly other side. Repeat until all 5 slices are cooked.
4. Garnish with fruits of choice. Serve with maple syrup on top.

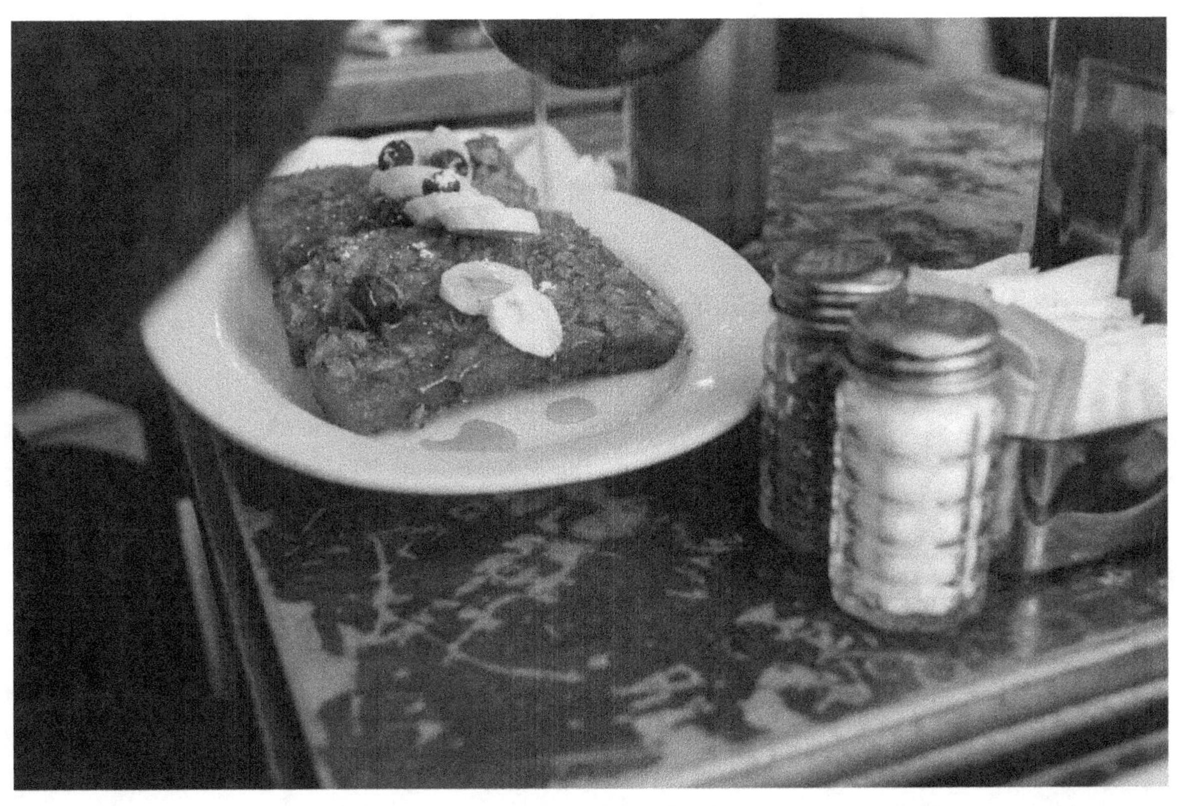

Cardamom Pancakes with Chocolate Buttons

Ingredients:

- 2 tablespoons maple syrup

- 2 tablespoons coconut oil, melted

- 1 cup all-purpose flour

- 1 cup coconut milk

- ¼ cup chocolate buttons

- 1 teaspoons apple cider vinegar

- ½ teaspoon baking powder

- ½ teaspoon baking soda

- ¼ teaspoon cardamom powder

- ¼ teaspoon vanilla extract

Directions:

1. Combine ingredients in large mixing bowl. Do not over mix. Lightly grease skillet with oil and set over medium heat.

2. Divide batter into 6 equal portions, about ¼ cup each. Pour into hot skillet. Flip when edges are set, and center is no longer runny. Do not press down on pancakes.

3. Plate. Add pinch of brown sugar on top for crunch (optional.) Serve.

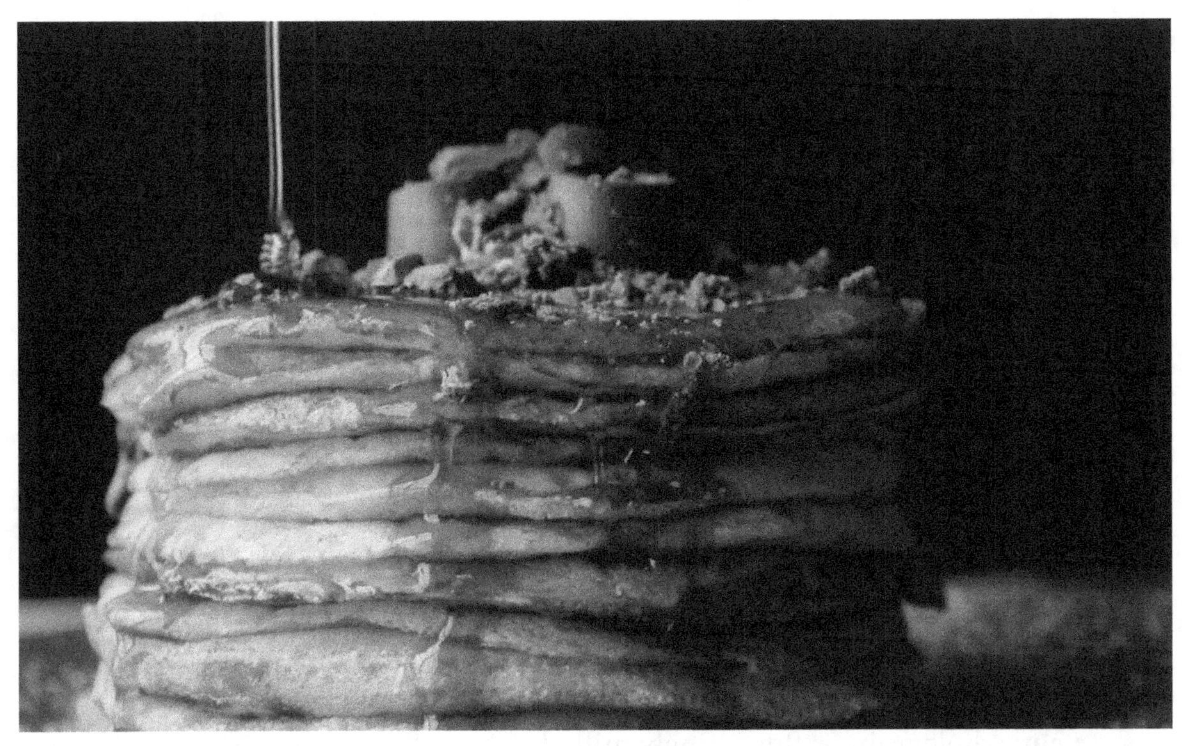

Pumpkin and Chocolate Pancakes

Ingredients:

- 2 tablespoons coconut oil, melted
- 2 tablespoons palm sugar, crumbled
- 1 tablespoon baking powder
- 1 teaspoon pumpkin pie spice
- 1 teaspoon vanilla extract
- ¼ teaspoon kosher salt
- 1 cup coconut milk
- 1 cup wholegrain or flour, finely milled
- ½ cup canned pumpkin puree
- ½ cup chocolate buttons

Directions:

1. Combine ingredients in large mixing bowl. Do not over mix. Lightly grease skillet with oil and set over medium heat.
2. Divide batter into 6 equal portions, about ¼ cup each. Pour into hot skillet. Flip when edges are set, and center is no longer runny. Do not press down on pancakes.
3. Plate. Add pinch of palm sugar on top for crunch (optional.) Serve.

Fruit-Filled Muffins

Ingredients:

- 2 cups flour

- 3 teaspoons baking powder

- ½ teaspoon salt

- Egg replacer

- ½ cup sweetener

- ¼ cup oil

- ¾ cup sour soy milk (add 1 teaspoon vinegar)

- 1 ½ cups frozen fruit of choice

Directions:

1. Preheat the oven to 350 degrees F.

2. Combine flour, baking powder, and salt in a bowl. Add egg replacer, sweetener, oil, sour milk, and fruit. Mix well.

3. Scoop into muffin tins. Bake for 30 minutes. Cool before serving.

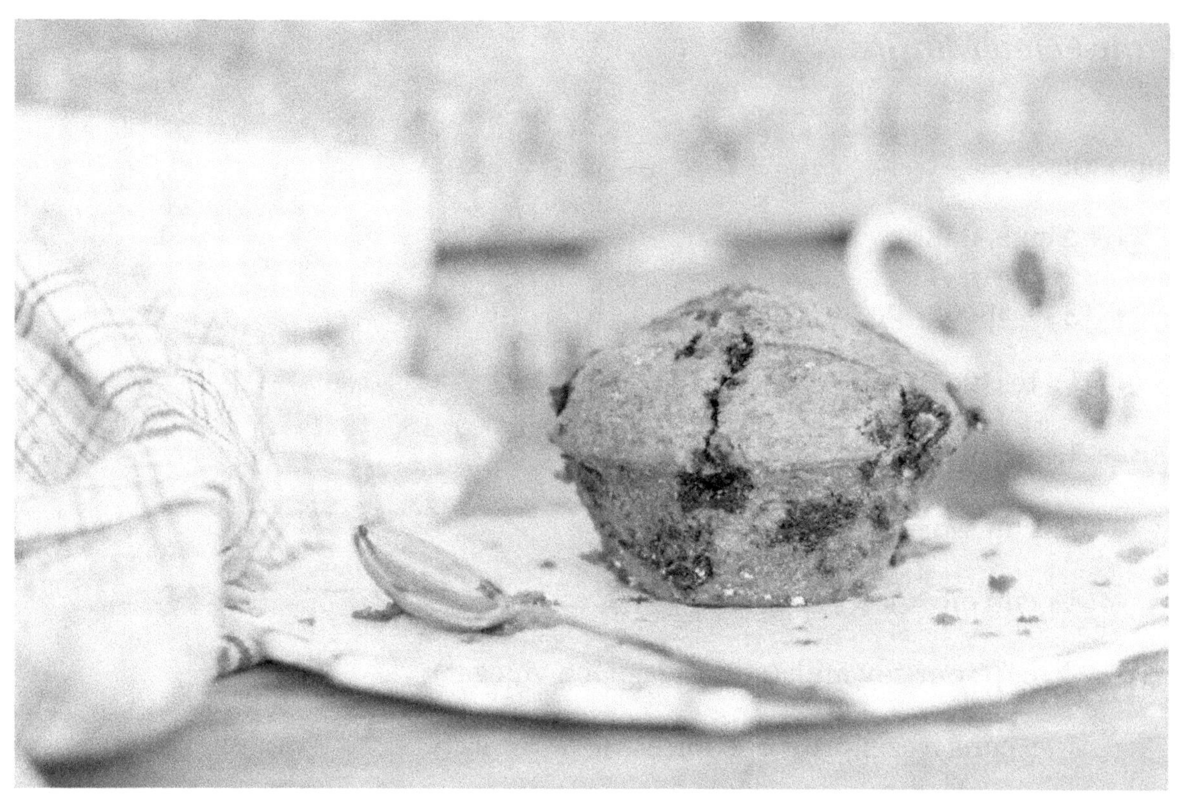

Almond Porridge with Fresh Fruits

Ingredients:

- 4 cups water

- ¾ cup steel-cut oats, gluten free

- 2 large bananas, mashed

- 1 vanilla pod, halved

- Dash of nutmeg

Garnishes

- 1 tablespoon almond slivers, toasted

- 1 kiwi fruit, diced

- 1 ripe mango, diced

- ¼ cup fresh blueberries

Directions:

1. Pour steel cut oats, vanilla pod, vanilla scrapings, and water in slow cooker set at low heat. Put lid on. Cook for 6 hours. Turn heat off. Stir in almond extract, bananas, and nutmeg.

2. Fish out and discard vanilla pod. Taste; add palm sugar only if needed. Ladle equal portions of porridge into individual bowls.

3. Garnish with blueberries, kiwifruit, mango, and almond slivers on top. Cool slightly before serving.

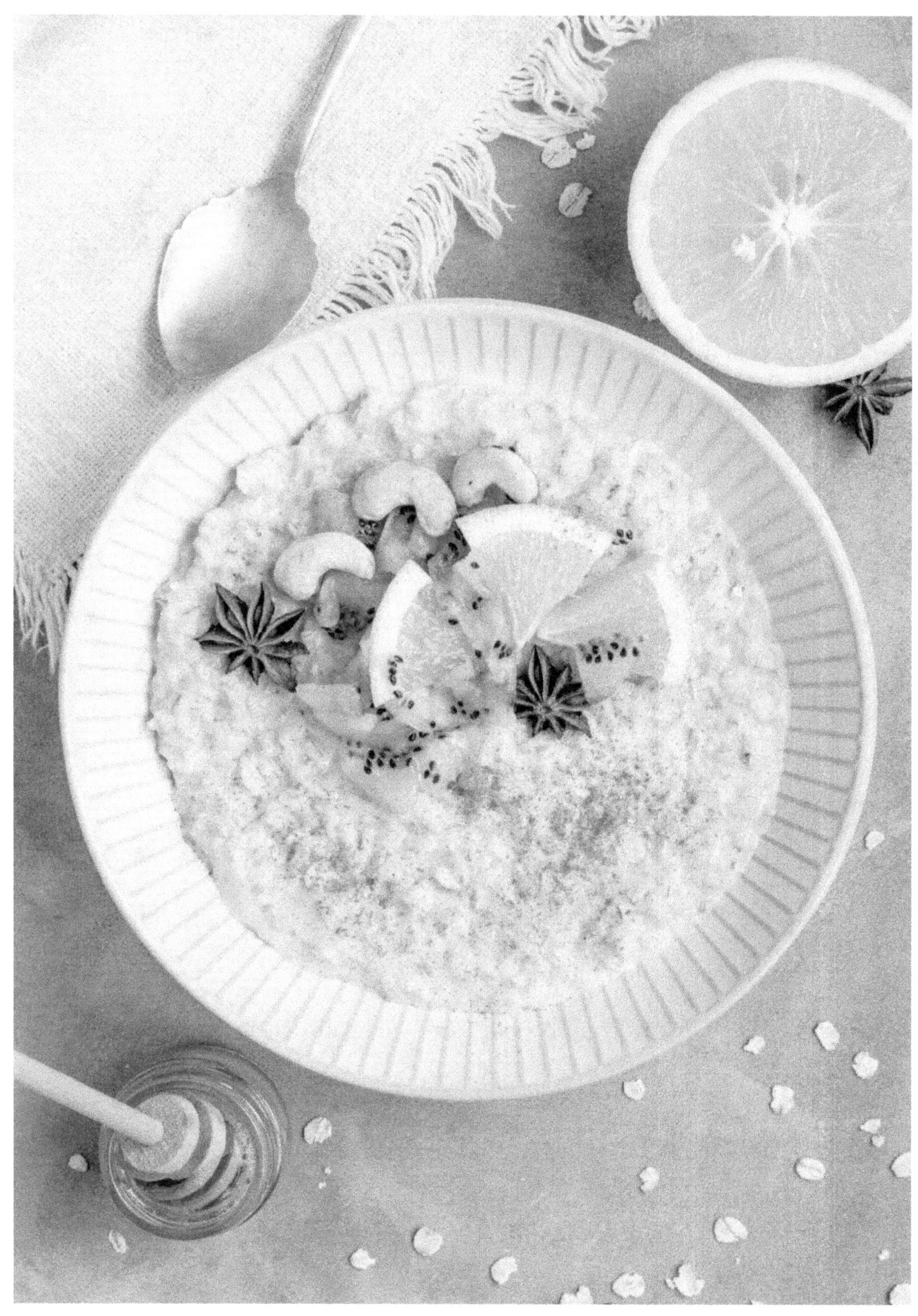

CHAPTER 4

Keto Vegan Lunch Recipes

Savory Roasted Cabbage

Ingredients:

- ¼ green cabbage head

- ¼ red cabbage head

- 1 ½ tablespoons olive oil

- 1 tablespoon balsamic vinegar

- Pinch of sea salt

- Pinch of white pepper

Directions:

1. Set the oven to 450 degrees F.

2. Chop the cabbages and arrange on a roasting pan. Drizzle the olive oil on top and toss well to coat. Season with salt and pepper, then toss again.

3. Roast for 8 to 10 minutes, stirring once every 3 minutes, until cabbage becomes slightly wilted.

4. Remove from the oven and drizzle the balsamic vinegar on top. Toss well, then serve right away.

Tofu Tacos

Ingredients:

- 6 organic corn tortillas, warmed
- ¾ tsp onion powder
- 7 oz extra firm organic tofu, drained
- ½ cup green onions, chopped
- ¼ cup hemp seeds
- ½ cup fresh cilantro leaves
- ¼ cup nutritional yeast
- 1 Tbsp. tahini
- ½ Tbsp. coconut oil
- 2 limes, sliced into wedges, for garnish

Directions:

1. Combine the tofu, tahini, onion powder, and nutritional yeast in a bowl. Mix well.
2. Place a cast iron skillet over medium high flame and heat through. Once hot, add the coconut oil, then sauté the tofu mixture until warmed through.
3. Turn off the heat and stir in the hemp seeds. Mix well, then transfer to a bowl.
4. Stuff the warmed tortillas with the tofu mixture, then top with cilantro leaves and green onion. Serve right with lime wedges.

Green Beans and Walnuts

Ingredients:

- ¾ lb. green beans, ends and strings removed
- 2 large garlic cloves, minced
- 1 large shallot, julienned
- 1 red chili, julienned
- 2 tablespoons mushroom stock, unsalted
- 1 tablespoon coconut oil
- 1 teaspoon fresh ginger, minced
- ¼ cup walnuts, garlic roasted, store-bought, chopped
- Pinch of kosher salt
- Pinch of white pepper

Directions:

1. Pour oil into wok set over medium heat. Add in and sauté garlic cloves, ginger, red chili, and shallot until limp and aromatic.
2. Pour in mushroom stock. Boil. Add in beans. Cook until these turns one shade brighter. Turn off heat. Sprinkle in walnuts.
3. Taste and season dish lightly. Divide into equal portions. Serve.

Brussels Sprouts with Lime Dip

Ingredients:

- 12 Brussels sprouts, halved

- Pinch of sea salt

- Pinch of black pepper

- 1 Tbsp. sunflower oil

For the Dip

- 1 tsp thyme leaves, minced

- 2 Tbsp. lemon juice, freshly squeezed

- 1 ½ Tbsp. pure maple syrup

- ½ Tbsp. hemp oil

Directions:

1. Set the oven to 500 degrees F.

2. Combine the ingredients for the dip in a bowl, mixing well. Set aside.

3. Place the Brussels sprouts on a rimmed baking sheet and drizzle the safflower or sunflower oil over them. Toss well to coat, then season with salt and pepper.

4. Add about half a tablespoon of water in the baking sheet with the Brussels sprouts, then cover the baking sheet with aluminum foil.

5. Roast for 10 minutes, then uncover the baking sheet and roast again for 10 minutes or until the Brussels sprouts are browned.

6. Remove the Brussels sprouts from the oven and add a tablespoon of the dip. Toss well to coat.

7. Skewer the Brussels sprouts through bamboo skewers. Serve on a plate with the dip in a bowl.

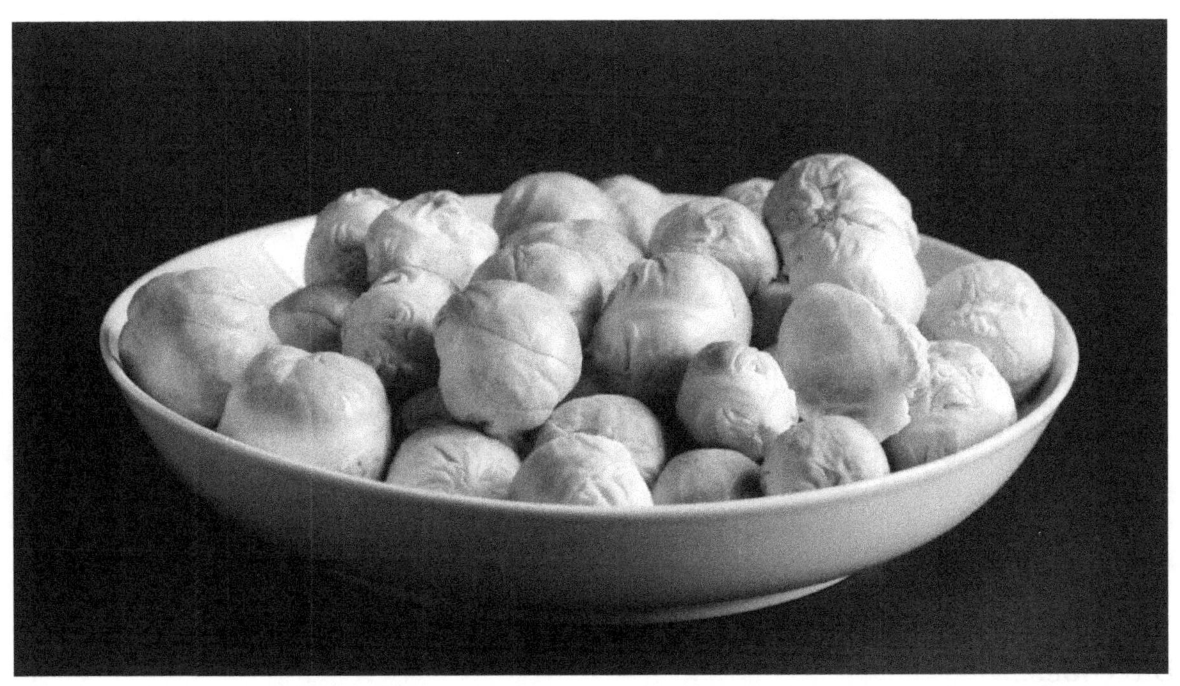

Lasagna Eggplant

Ingredients:

- 2 eggplant
- ½ cup baby spinach
- 2 cups tomato sauce, low-sodium
- ½ cup ricotta cheese, fat-free
- 1/3 cup Parmesan cheese, grated

Directions:

1. Set the oven to 450 F.
2. Chop eggplant to quarter-inch thick pieces after slicing lengthwise. Transfer onto a cooking spray-coated cookie sheet.
3. Place in the oven to roast for 20 minutes or until tender, making sure to turn after 10 minutes. Once done, take out of the oven and set on a cooling rack. Meanwhile, turn down the heat to 350 F.
4. Fill a microwaveable dish with the baby spinach. Sprinkle with water and cook until wilted before squeezing dry.
5. Fill the bottom of a baking dish with a portion of tomato sauce. Top with a portion each of eggplant slices, spinach, and ricotta cheese. Repeat with the remaining tomato sauce, eggplant slices, spinach, and ricotta cheese.
6. Top with freshly grated Parmesan cheese. Place in the oven to bake for about twenty to twenty-five minutes or until the cheese is bubbling. Serve.

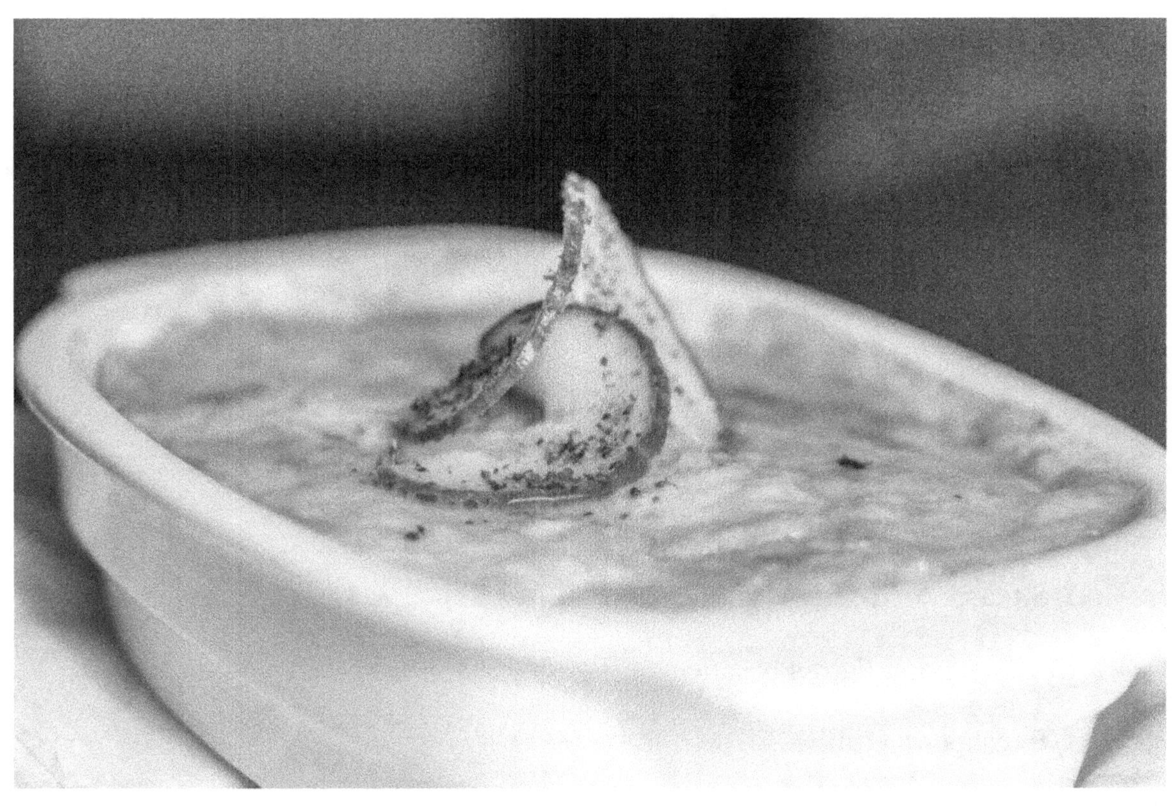

Tofu Tacos

Ingredients:

- 1 teaspoons olive oil
- ½ cup firm tofu, crumbled
- ½ onion, chopped
- ½ teaspoon garlic powder
- ½ tablespoon chilli power
- 1/8 teaspoon dried oregano
- ½ tablespoon light soy sauce
- 1/8 teaspoon cumin
- 3 corn tortillas
- 2 tablespoons tomato sauce
- 1 cup lettuce, shredded
- ¼ cup tomato, chopped
- ¼ cup green onion
- 2 ½ tablespoon salsa

Directions:

1. Place a frying pan over medium flame and heat through. Once hot, add the oil and swirl to coat.

2. Saute onion until translucent. Stir in tofu, onion, garlic powder, chili powder, oregano, soy sauce, and cumin. Stir until the tofu is crumbly.

3. Pour tomato sauce. Reduce to low flame. Sauté until liquid has evaporated.

4. Reheat tortillas in a dry, nonstick frying pan. Transfer to a plate. Spoon tofu filling in the center and add lettuce, tomato, green onion, and salsa. Roll up and serve.

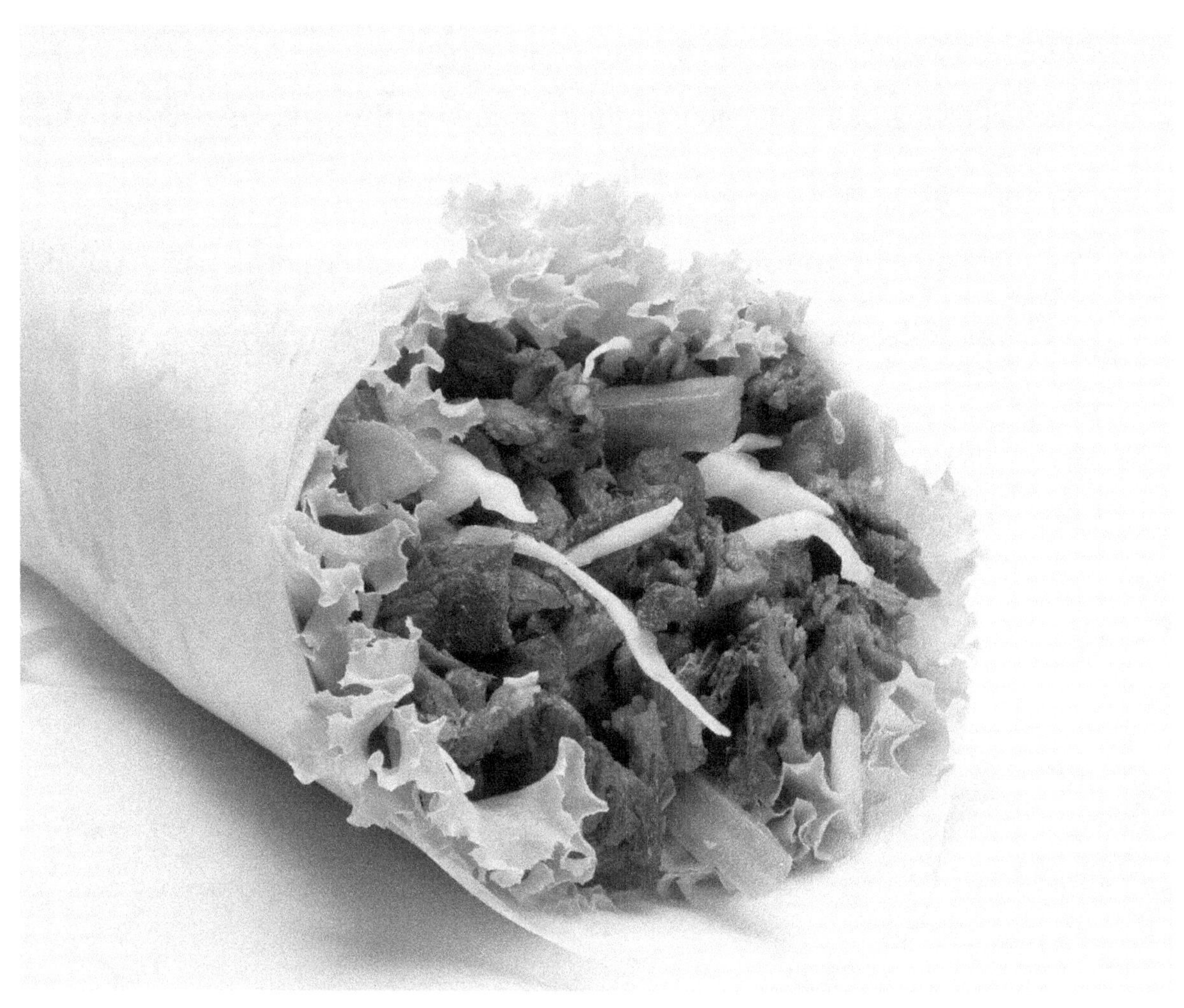

Bean Burrito

Ingredients:

- 2 whole wheat tortillas
- 1 can nonfat beans
- 1/2 cup romaine lettuce, shredded
- 1 tomato, chopped
- ¼ cup salsa
- 1 green onion, chopped

Directions:

1. Heat tortillas on a pan set over medium heat.
2. Divide beans among tortillas. Add lettuce on top. Tip in tomatoes, salsa, and green onion.
3. Fold tortillas. Serve.

Veggie Salad in Soy Vinaigrette

Ingredients:

- ¼ cup roasted walnuts, chopped

For the Vinaigrette

- 3 tablespoons light soy sauce

- 2 tablespoons extra virgin olive oil

- 1 tablespoon palm sugar, crumbled

- 1 ½ teaspoon chili oil

- 1 teaspoon garlic, grated

- 1 teaspoon ginger, grated

- 1 teaspoon sesame oil

- ½ cup rice wine vinegar

- Pinch of Himalayan pink salt

- Pinch of white pepper

For the Salad

- 6 cups napa cabbage, julienned

- 2 cups red cabbage, julienned

- 1 cup carrot, julienned

- ½ cup leeks, minced

- 1 can Mandarin oranges in water, drained

- 1 can sliced water chestnuts, drained

Directions:

1. Combine vinaigrette ingredients in a bowl; whisk. Taste; adjust seasoning if needed. Set aside.

2. Place salad ingredients in a bowl; drizzle in half of vinaigrette. Toss to combine. Serve equal portions into plates. Drizzle in remaining vinaigrette; sprinkle garlic-roasted walnuts on top. Serve.

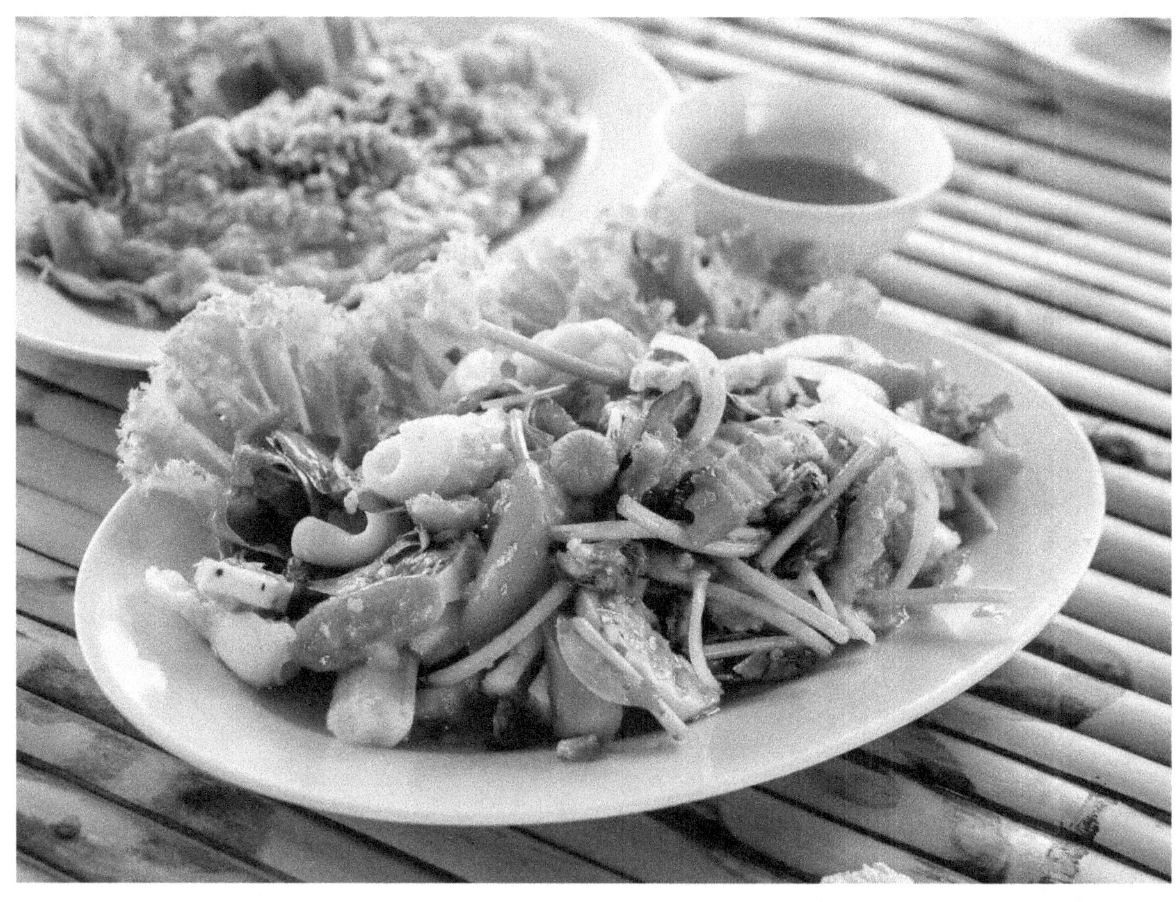

Veggie Pitas

Ingredients:

- 2 vegan burger patties
- 2 whole pitas, halved
- 4 cups romaine lettuce, chopped
- ½ cup shredded carrot
- 4 plum tomatoes, thinly sliced
- 2 tablespoons spicy mustard

Directions:

1. Heat vegan burger patties based on the manufacturer's instructions. Halve and set aside.
2. Heat the halved pitas in the microwave. Spread spicy mustard inside.
3. Stuff with burger patties, lettuce, carrot, and tomatoes. Serve.

Green Salad with Basil Dressing

Ingredients:

- 1 head iceberg lettuce, torn, chilled well prior to use

- 1 cucumber, sliced into thin half-moons

For the Dressing

- 3 teaspoon red wine vinegar

- 3 teaspoon extra virgin olive oil

- 1 teaspoon Dijon mustard

- ½ teaspoon dried basil leaves

- 1 garlic clove, minced

- Pinch of kosher salt

- Pinch of white pepper

Directions:

1. Pour dressing ingredients into small bottle with tight fitting lid. Seal and shake bottle until dressing emulsifies.

2. Place remaining ingredients into salad bowl; drizzle in dressing. Toss to combine. Place equal portions into bowls. Serve.

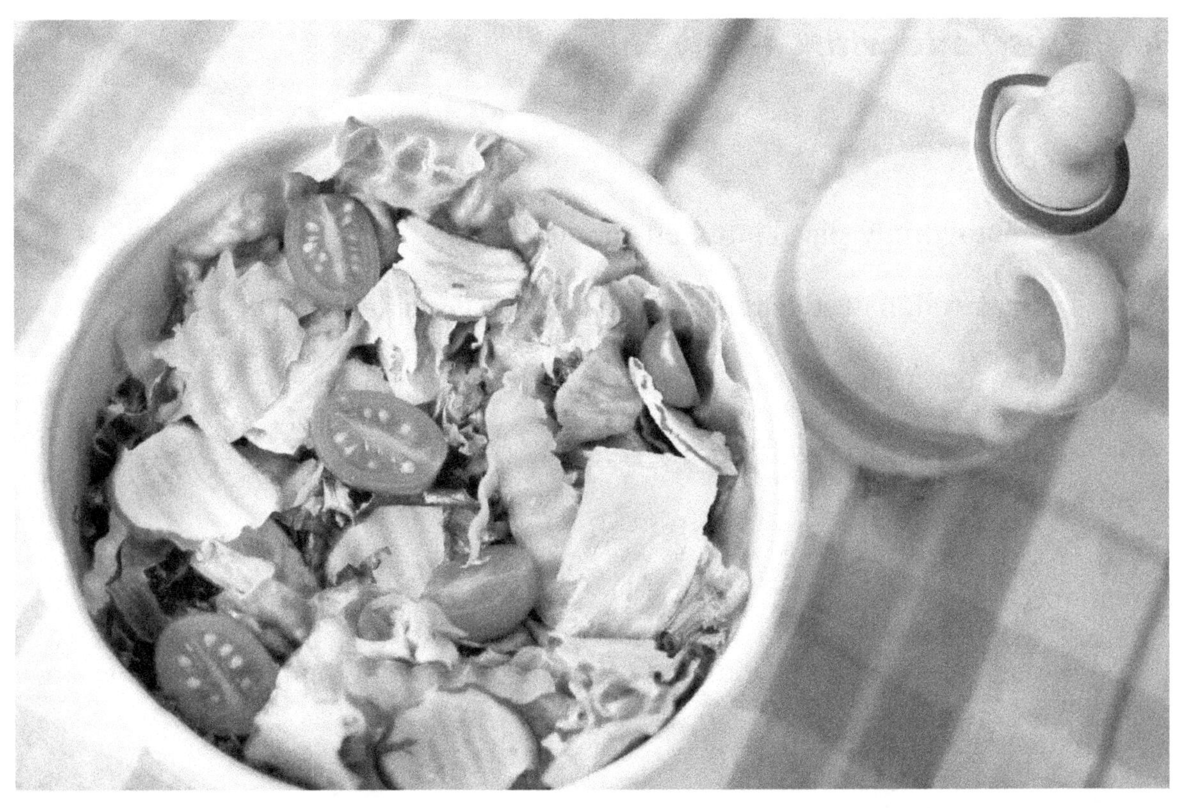

Basil Bruschetta with Cashew Cheese

Ingredients:

- 1 tomato, thinly sliced into half-moons
- 1 Kaiser roll, halved lengthwise, toasted on cut sides
- 1 tablespoon Basil Pesto Sauce
- 1 tablespoon Cashew Cheese

Directions:

1. Spread/place equal portion of pesto sauce first, and then tomato slices on cut sides of bread roll.
2. Drizzle cashew cheese on top.
3. Heat bruschetta in toaster oven until warmed through. Serve while warm.

Boodles (Broccoli Stem Noodles)

Ingredients:

- 2 large fresh broccoli stems, trimmed well to make scraping easier

- Pinch of kosher salt

Directions:

1. Make deep scores spaced ⅛-inch apart on one side of broccoli stem. Using vegetable peeler, scrape cut side of vegetable repeatedly until you have a pile of noodles; make sure that you use long strokes. Discard the rest.

2. Place vegetables and salt into colander. Toss well to combine. Let vegetables "sweat" and drain for 30 minutes. Shake off excess moisture.

3. Layer boodles on tea towel; roll tightly to remove more moisture and salt.

4. Remove vegetable noodles from tea towel. Do not rinse. Use as needed.

Squadles (Squash Noodles)

Ingredients:

- 2 large fresh parsnip, peeled

- Pinch of kosher salt

Directions:

1. Make deep scores spaced ⅛-inch apart on one side of squash. Using vegetable peeler, scrape cut side of the vegetable repeatedly until you have a pile of noodles; make sure that you use long strokes. Discard the rest.

2. Mix and toss vegetables and salt into colander. Let vegetables "sweat" and drain for 30 minutes. Shake off excess moisture.

3. Layer squadles on tea towel; roll tightly to remove more moisture and salt. Remove vegetable noodles from tea towel. Use as needed.

Smooth and Spicy Veggie Soup

Ingredients:

- 6 cups mushroom stock

- 2 cups raw cashew nuts, whole

- 4 garlic cloves, minced

- 2 red bell pepper, deseeded, diced

- 2 carrots, peeled, diced

- 1 celery, diced

- 1 sweet potato, cubed

- 1 large onion, minced

- 1 bird's eye chili, deseeded, optional

- 1 tablespoon olive oil

- ¼ teaspoon cayenne pepper

- ¼ teaspoon red pepper flakes

- ¼ teaspoon Himalayan pinks salt

- Pinch of white pepper

Directions:

1. Pour oil into Dutch oven set over medium heat. Sauté garlic and onion until limp and transparent; add in remaining ingredients. Boil.

2. Reduce heat to lowest setting. Cook until vegetables are tender, about 30 minutes. Turn off heat; process soup until smooth using an immersion blender.

3. Taste; adjust seasoning if needed. Ladle soup into bowls. Serve.

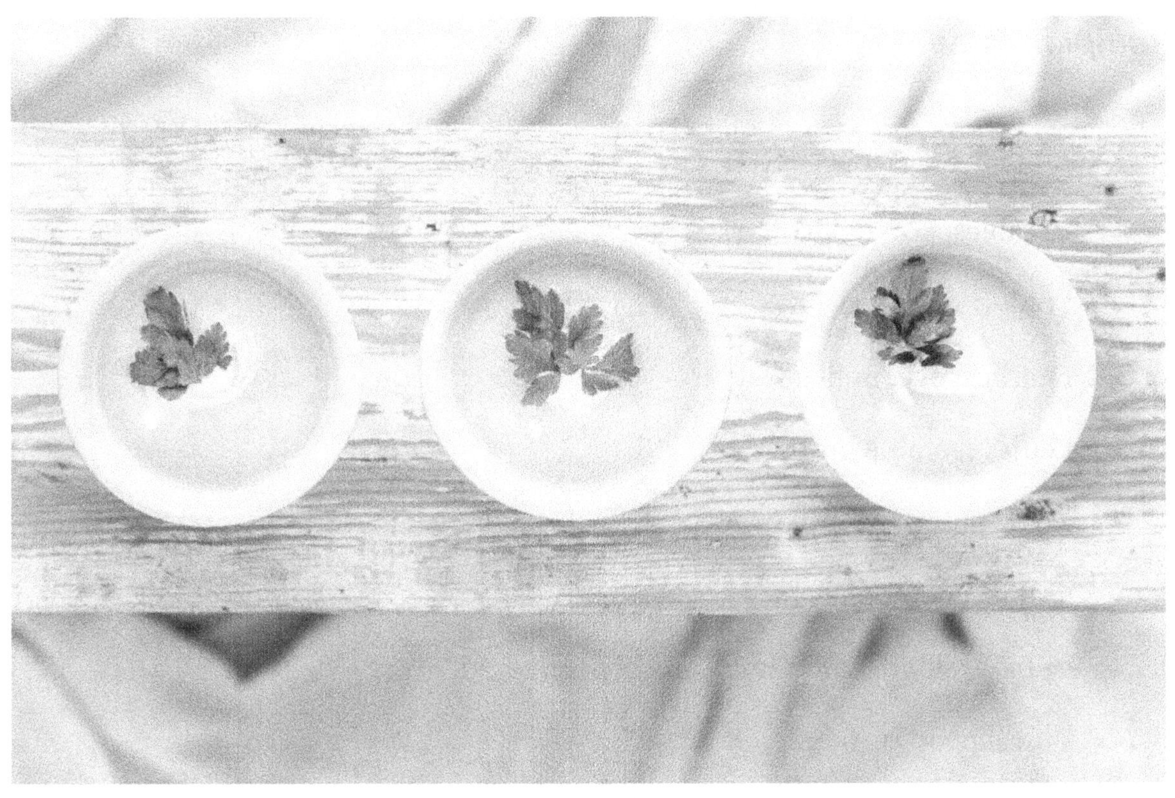

Pumpkin Stew

Ingredients:

- ½ tablespoon olive oil

- 1 onion, chopped

- 1 garlic clove, minced

- 1 cup vegetable broth

- 7.5 oz pureed pumpkin

- 1 tablespoon honey

- ½ tablespoon lemon juice, freshly squeezed

- ¼ teaspoon turmeric

- ¼ teaspoon mustard seeds

- ¼ teaspoon cumin

- 1/8 teaspoon cinnamon

- 1/3 teaspoon fine sea salt

- ¼ teaspoon ground ginger

- 1cup soy milk

Directions:

1. Place a saucepan over medium flame and heat through. Add the oil and swirl to coat.

2. Sauté the onion and garlic until tender. Stir in the spices and salt until ragrant. Stir in the broth, pumpkin, honey, and lemon juice.

3. Simmer for 8 minutes, then serve

CHAPTER 5

Vegan Keto Dinner Recipes

Chili and Bean Rice

Ingredients:

- 3 cups white long-grained rice, cooked

- 2 jalapeno pepper, minced

- 1 can black beans, rinsed, drained

- ⅛ teaspoon chili powder

- 1/8 teaspoon cumin powder

- ⅛ teaspoon garlic powder

- ⅛ teaspoon onion powder

- ⅛ teaspoon kosher salt

- 2 cups mushroom stock

- ¼ cup fresh cilantro, minced

Directions:

1. Except for cilantro, pour ingredients into rice cooker. Pour stock until liquid reaches 4-cup line of pot. Stir; secure lid. Press cook; wait for machine to automatically shift to warm. Turn off heat.

2. Ladle recommended portions into bowls. Serve with a pinch of cilantro on top.

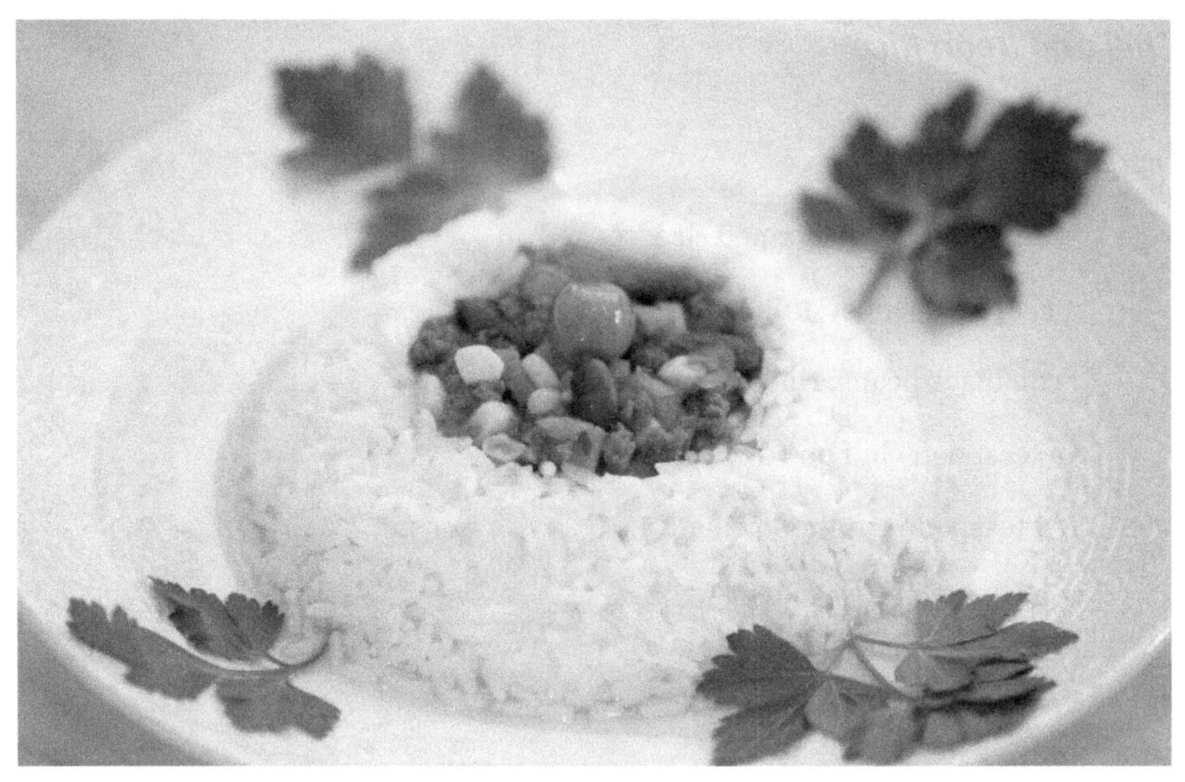

Breaded Baby Carrots

Ingredients:

- 1-pound baby carrots

- 1 cup almond flour, finely milled

- 1 cup almond milk

- 1 cup panko breading

- olive oil for shallow frying

- Pinch of kosher salt

- Pinch of white pepper

- Dash of Spanish paprika

Directions:

1. Pour oil into non-stick skillet set over medium heat. Meanwhile, place flour, milk, and *panko* breading into 3 different shallow bowls.

2. Dredge one baby carrot in flour first, and then into the milk; coat generously with *panko* breading. Repeat step until all baby corn are breaded. Fry these in oil until crisp and golden brown. Drain on paper towels.

3. Just before serving, season well with salt and paprika.

Bean Casserole

Ingredients:

- 4 cups mushroom stock

- 1 cup dried black beans, rinsed, drained

- 1 cup dried pinto beans, rinsed, drained

- 1 carrot, diced

- 1 shallot, minced

- 1 red bell pepper, diced

- 1 teaspoon oregano powder

- 1 can diced and peeled tomatoes

- Pinch of kosher salt

- Pinch of white pepper

Directions:

1. Except for canned tomatoes, pour ingredients into slow cooker set at medium heat. Stir; secure lid.

2. Cook for 6 hours, or until beans are fork tender. Turn off heat. Stir in tomatoes. Let dish rest for 15 minutes, covered.

3. Ladle recommended serving into bowls. Serve.

Broccoli and Cauliflower Stir-Fry

Ingredients:

- 2 garlic cloves, minced

- 1 shallot, minced

- 1 red bell pepper, cubed

- 2 heads broccoli, sliced into bite-sized florets

- 2 heads cauliflower, sliced into bite-sized florets

- 2 tablespoons vegetable stock

- 1 tablespoons coconut oil

- Pinch of kosher salt

- Pinch of white pepper

Directions:

1. Pour oil into wok set over medium heat. Add in and sauté garlic and shallot until limp and aromatic. Add in remaining ingredients.

2. Cook only until broccoli turns a shade brighter. This will allow veggies to remain crisp but tender. Turn off heat. Taste; season lightly.

3. Divide into equal portions. Serve.

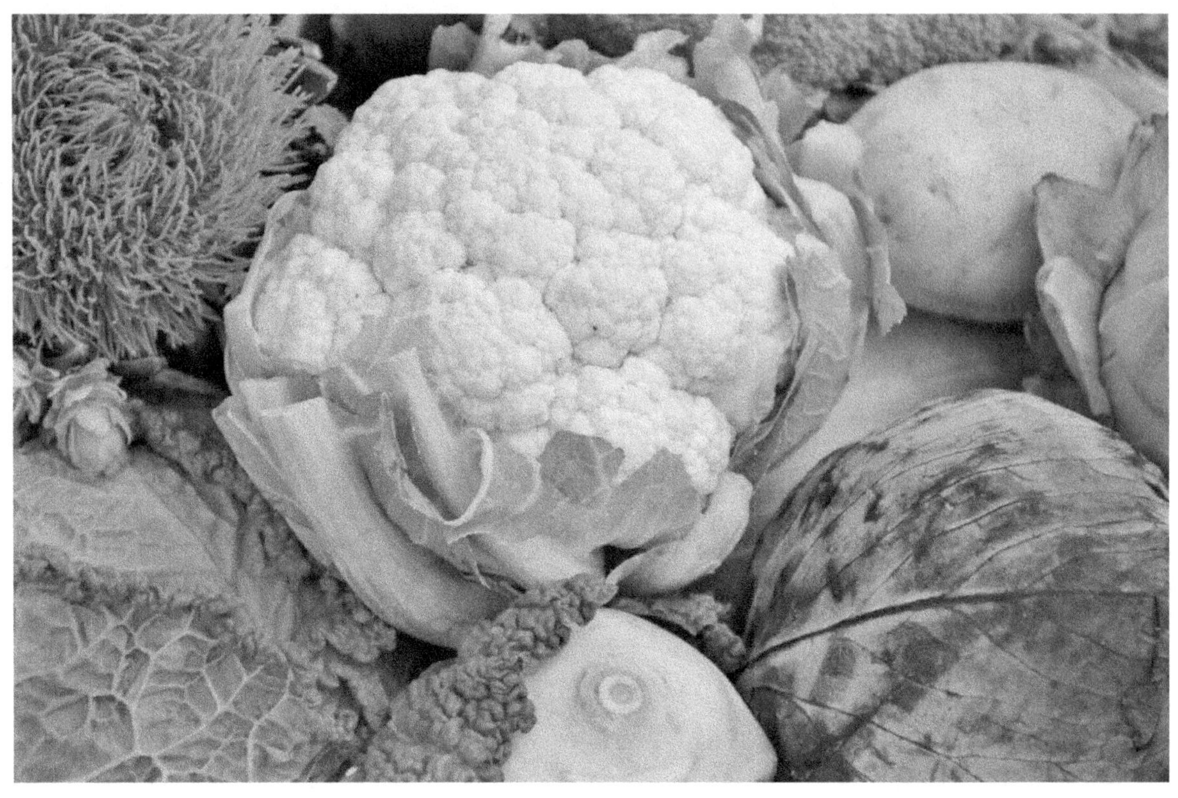

Chop Suey with Straw Mushrooms

Ingredients:

- 2 garlic cloves, minced

- 1 carrot, sliced into ⅛-inch thick half-moons

- 1 cauliflower, sliced into florets

- 1 shallot, minced

- 2 tablespoons vegetable stock

- 1 tablespoon coconut oil

- 1 cup snow peas, rinsed, drained

- 1 can straw mushrooms, rinsed, drained

- Pinch of kosher salt

- Pinch of white pepper

Directions:

1. Pour oil into wok set over medium heat. Add in and sauté garlic cloves and shallot until limp and aromatic.

2. Add in carrots and cauliflower; stir-fry for 3 minutes. Pour in vegetable stock. Boil. Add in mushrooms and snow peas. Cook until peas turn one shade brighter. Turn off heat.

3. Taste and season dish lightly. Divide into equal portions. Serve.

Courgette Pasta with Mixed Greens and Fruits Salad

Ingredients:

- 1 package courgettes pasta

- 1 garlic clove

- 1 cup fresh basil

- 1 tsp. ground pepper

- 1/2 cup pine nuts

- 1/3 cup red wine vinegar

- 1 tsp. mustard

- Mixed salad greens, for garnish

- Grape tomatoes, for garnish

- Yellow tomatoes, for garnish

- 3/4 cup olive oil

Directions:

1. In a medium pot, add water and boil the small pasta shells until al dente.

2. To prepare the dressing, whisk the vinegar, oil and pepper in a medium bowl.

3. Once the pasta is cooked, add the vinaigrette dressing over it and add the basil, pine nuts and cheese.

4. In a plate, add grape tomatoes, mixed salad greens and yellow tomatoes.

5. Toss all the salad ingredients and serve in individual plates, garnish with grape tomatoes, yellow tomatoes and mixed salad greens.

Baked Onion Rings

Ingredients:

- 3 sweet onions, sliced into thick rings

- 1 ½ cups plain breadcrumbs

- 1 ½ cups all-purpose flour

- 1 ¼ cups water

- 1 ¼ tsp sea salt

- 1 ½ Tbsp. olive oil

Directions:

1. Set the oven to 450 degrees F.

2. Lightly coat a baking sheet with the olive oil cooking spray. Set aside.

3. In a bowl, combine ¾ teaspoon of salt with the flour. Stir in the tonic water until a smooth batter form.

4. In a dish, combine the remaining salt with the canola oil and breadcrumbs.

5. Dip each onion ring into the batter, then dredge in the breadcrumb mixture until thoroughly coated.

6. Lay the onion rings on the prepared baking sheet, then transfer to the freezer and freeze for at least 20 minutes to firm up the batter.

7. Bake the frozen onion rings for 10 minutes per side, or until golden brown.

8. Set on a cooling rack and let stand for 5 minutes, then serve.

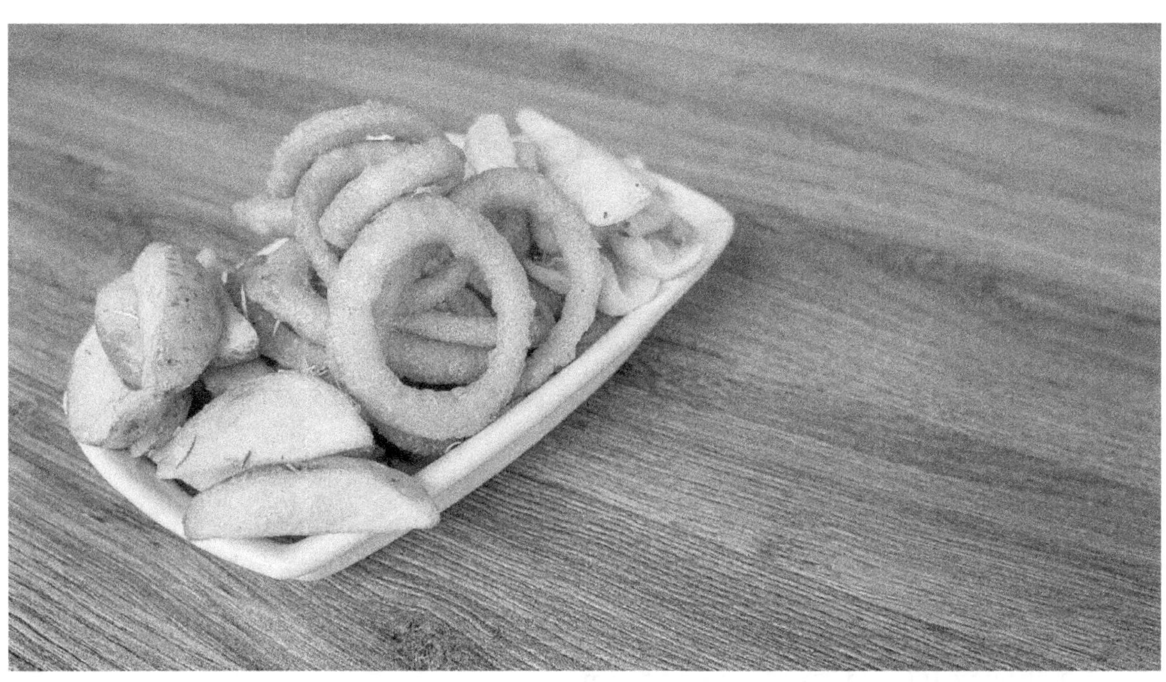

Spicy Stuffed Bell Peppers

Ingredients:

- 4 bell peppers, roasted
- 4 garlic cloves, minced
- 1 yellow onion, minced
- 2 cups cauliflower rice
- 1 carrot, minced
- 1 zucchini, minced
- 2 cups vegetable broth, low sodium
- 1 ½ cups canned chickpeas
- 3 tsp ground coriander
- 1 ½ tsp sea salt
- 1/3 tsp ground black pepper
- 1 ½ tsp paprika
- 1 ½ tsp ground cinnamon
- 1 ½ tsp sea salt
- 4 ½ Tbsp. tomato paste
- 3 tsp hot chili paste
- ¾ tsp ground cumin
- 3 tsp olive oil

Directions:

1. Slice the tops off the bell peppers and discard the seeds. Set aside.

2. Sauté the vegetables in the olive oil in a saucepan over medium flame, then stir in the spices, salt, and pepper.

3. Add the cauliflower rice, chili paste, tomato paste, and vegetable broth, stirring well. Fold in the chickpeas and cover.

4. Cook until the cauliflower rice has absorbed the broth.

5. Stuff the mixture into the roasted bell peppers, then serve right away.

Spiced Cherry Tomatoes and Cucumber Salad

Ingredients:

- 6 cherry tomatoes, quartered
- 2 cucumbers, unpeeled, thinly sliced
- 1 bird's eye chili, minced
- 1 head escarole, torn
- 1 cup heaping cos lettuce, torn
- ½ cup black olives in oil, drained

Dressing

- ½ cup basil leaves, julienned
- 1 tablespoon balsamic vinegar
- 1 tablespoon apple cider vinegar
- 1 tablespoon lemon juice, freshly squeezed
- 1 tablespoon extra-virgin olive oil
- ⅛ teaspoon sea salt
- Pinch of black pepper

Directions:

1. Whisk dressing ingredients in a bowl until salt dissolves. Taste; adjust seasoning if needed.
2. Place remaining ingredients in a bowl; drizzle in vinegar mix. Toss gently to combine. Spoon equal amounts into individual serving bowls; serve

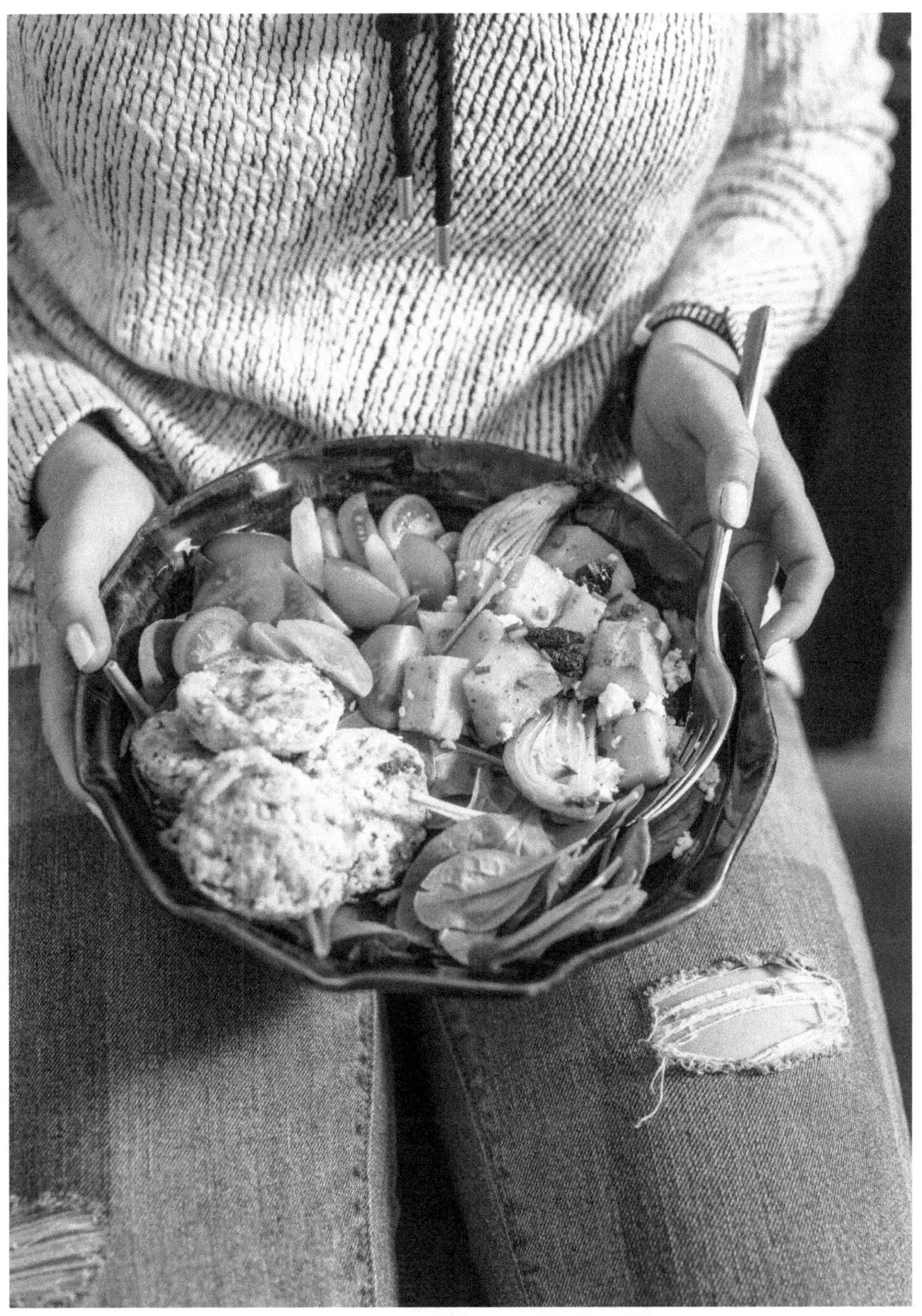

Cauliflower Pop

Ingredients:

- 2 cauliflower heads, sliced into bite-sized florets
- Pinch of sea salt, to taste
- olive oil, for drizzling

Directions:

1. Preheat oven to 425°F/215°C. Line 2 baking sheets with aluminum foil.
2. Place cauliflower on baking sheets. Drizzle in oil; season lightly with paprika and sea salt.
3. Bake an hour; flip veggies over 3 to 4 times after the first 20 minutes. Cool slightly before serving. Taste; sprinkle in more seasonings only if needed. Serve.

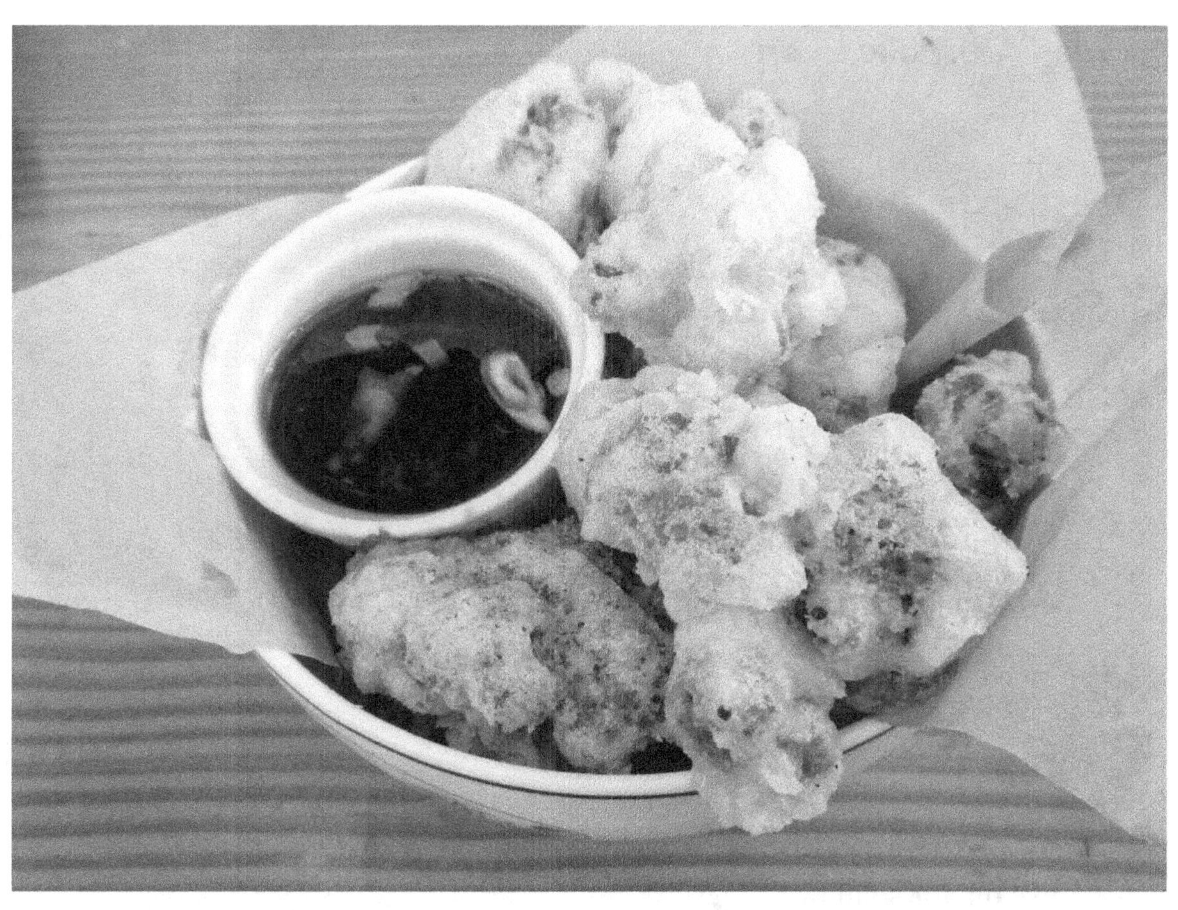

Breaded Artichoke Hearts

Ingredients:

Artichokes

- 1 lb. fresh artichoke hearts, quartered
- ½ cup ground flaxseed and 3 tablespoons water to serve as egg replacement
- 1 cup almond meal
- 1 cup almond flour, finely milled
- Pinch of sea salt
- Pinch of white pepper
- ½ lemon, sliced into wedges
- olive oil, for shallow frying

Directions:

1. Pour small amount of oil into non-stick skillet set over medium heat. Lightly season veggies with salt and pepper, before dredging in almond flour first, and then into flaxseed, and into almond meal; shake off excess starch.
2. Carefully slide breaded veggies into oil; fry until crisp and golden, flipping often. Drain on paper towels.
3. Serve equal portions on plates with wedge of lime. Squeeze lime juice over vegetables just before serving.

Spicy Tofu Paella

Ingredients:

- 1 package spicy marinated tofu, diced
- 2 green onions, thinly sliced
- 2 garlic cloves, minced
- ½ cup carrot, diced
- 4 oz sliced cremini mushrooms
- 7 oz canned tomatoes, drained, chopped
- 1 cup vegetable broth, low sodium
- ½ cup peas
- 1 cup cauliflower rice
- 2 Tbsp. lemon juice, freshly squeezed
- 1 Tbsp. olive oil
- Pinch of sea salt
- Pinch of ground black pepper

Directions:

1. Place a wok over medium high flame and heat through. Once hot, add the oil and swirl to coat.

2. Sauté the diced tofu until golden brown, then stir in the mushrooms. Sauté until tender.

3. Add the carrots, garlic, and tomatoes. Sauté for 2 minutes. Pour the vegetable broth and cauliflower rice. Bring to a boil. Once boiling, reduce to medium low flame.

4. Cover the wok. Simmer for 30 minutes.

5. Fold in the peas and steam for 1 minute. Turn off the heat, then fold in the green onions and lemon juice. Season with salt and pepper. Serve.

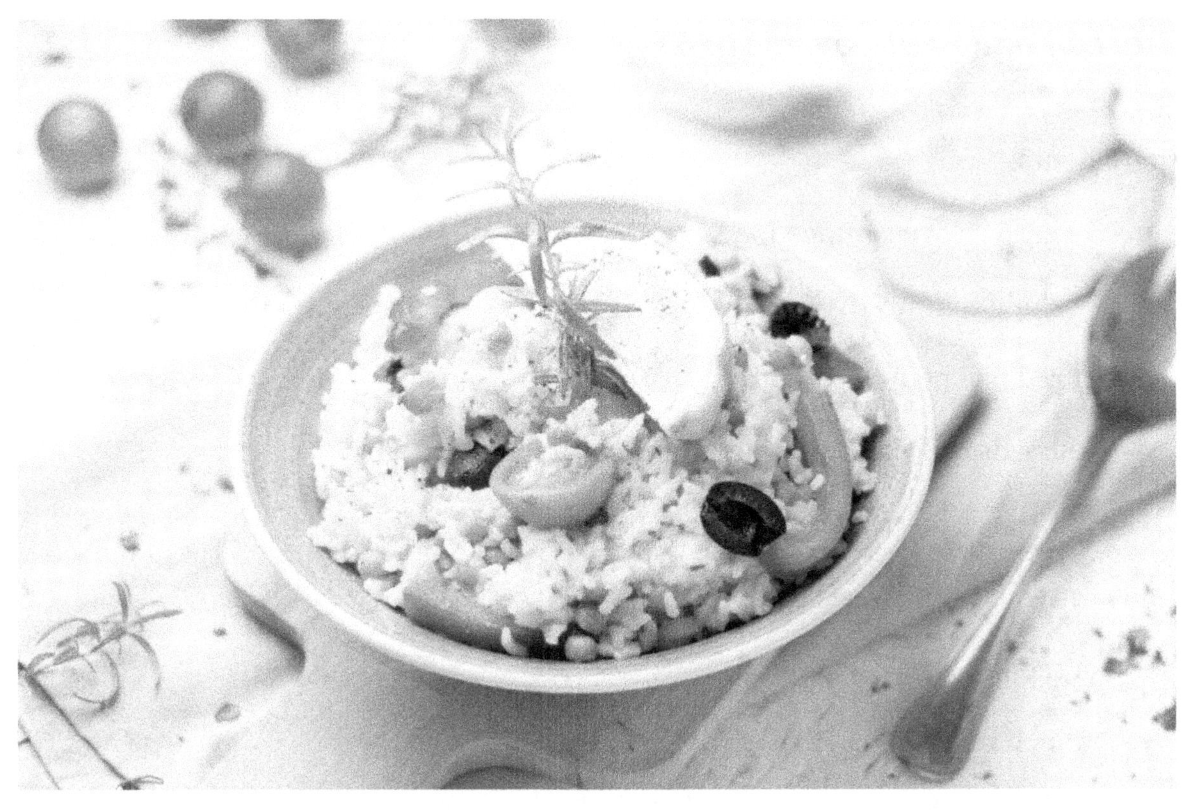

Broccoli and Cauliflower Stir-Fry

Ingredients:

- 2 garlic cloves, minced

- 1 shallot, minced

- 1 red bell pepper, cubed

- 2 heads broccoli, sliced into bite-sized florets

- 2 heads cauliflower, sliced into bite-sized florets

- 2 tablespoons vegetable stock

- 1 tablespoons coconut oil

- Pinch of kosher salt

- Pinch of white pepper

Directions:

1. Pour oil into wok set over medium heat. Add in and sauté garlic and shallot until limp and aromatic. Add in remaining ingredients.

2. Cook only until broccoli turns a shade brighter. This will allow veggies to remain crisp but tender. Turn off heat. Taste; season lightly.

3. Divide into equal portions. Serve.

Lentil with Butternut Squash Soup

Ingredients:

- 4 cups mushroom stock
- 1 cup green lentils, rinsed
- 2 garlic cloves, minced
- 1 carrot, minced
- 1 white onion, minced
- ½ butternut squash, diced
- 1 tablespoon olive oil
- 1 can tomatoes, diced
- ½ teaspoon dried thyme
- Pinch of kosher salt

Directions:

1. Pour oil into Dutch oven set over medium heat. When oil is hot enough, add in and sauté onion and garlic until limp and aromatic.

2. Add in remaining ingredients. Stir. Bring soup to a boil. Secure lid. Turn down heat. Simmer for 30 minutes. Turn off heat.

3. Taste; adjust seasoning, if needed. Cool slightly before serving.

Celery and Kale Tiger Salad

Ingredients:

For the Dressing

- 2 drops chili oil, optional

- 2 garlic cloves, crushed

- 1 banana chili, roughly chopped

- 1 green chili, roughly chopped

- 1 tablespoon palm sugar, crumbled

- ½ cup lime juice, freshly squeezed

- Pinch of kosher salt

- Pinch of white pepper

For the Salad

- 6 cups kale leaves, shredded

- ½ cup basil leaves, torn

- ½ cup cilantro leaves, torn

- ½ cup mint leaves, torn

- ½ cup pumpkin seeds, roasted

- 2 celery stalks, minced

- 2 leeks, minced

Directions:

1. Pour dressing ingredients in a small bottle with tight-fitting lid. Shake well until salt and sugar dissolves. Taste; adjust seasoning if needed. Set aside.

2. Except for pumpkin seeds, place salad ingredients in large bowl. Drizzle in half of dressing; toss well.

3. Ladle equal portions into plates. Add more dressing if desired; sprinkle pumpkin seeds on top. Serve immediately.

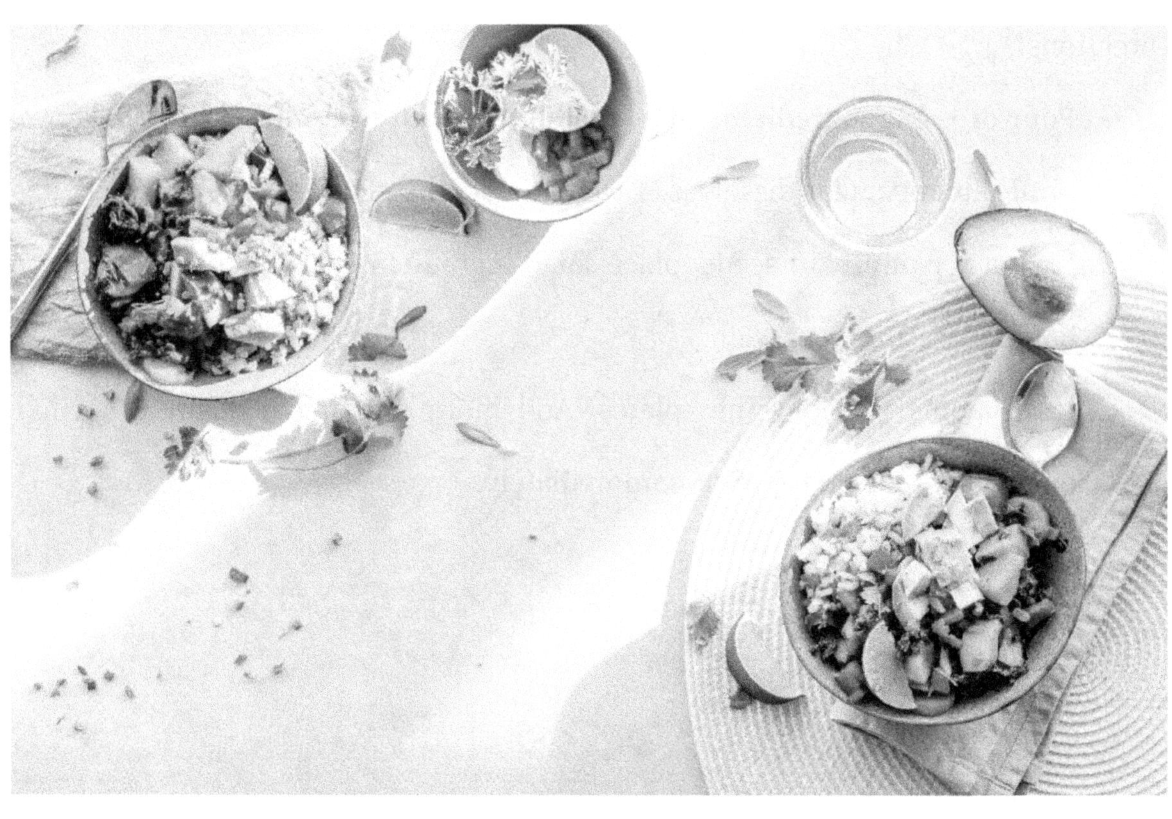

Three Mushroom Quinoa Congee

Ingredients:

- 6¼ cups water
- ¼ cup quinoa
- 2 tablespoons coconut oil, divided
- 1 tablespoon fresh ginger, grated
- 2 shallots, minced
- 2 garlic cloves, grated
- 1 can straw mushrooms, rinsed, drained well
- ½ pound fresh portabella mushrooms, diced
- ¼ pound dried shiitake mushrooms
- Pinch of sea salt
- Pinch of white pepper
- 1 lime, sliced into wedges
- ¼ cup fresh chives, minced
- red pepper flakes

Directions:

1. Soak dried shiitake mushrooms in water for at least 1 hour before using. Discard tough stems; dice caps. Place mushrooms into slow cooker set at low heat. Except for inch of water containing debris, pour mushrooms' soaking liquid into slow cooker as well.

2. Pour 1 Tbsp. oil into large skillet set over medium heat. Stir-fry diced portabella mushrooms until brown. Push mushrooms to one side of pan.

3. Pour in remaining oil; sauté shallots, garlic, and ginger until limp and aromatic; pour into slow cooker. Except for garnishes, pour in remaining ingredients; stir. Put lid on. Cook for 6 hours. Turn off heat. Taste; adjust seasoning if needed.

4. Ladle congee into individual bowls. Garnish with chives and pepper flakes. Serve with wedge of lime on the side. Squeeze lime juice into congee just before eating.

Zucchini and Tomato Curry

Ingredients:

- 1 tablespoon olive oil

- 1 red onion, diced

- 2 garlic cloves, minced

- 1 teaspoon ginger, freshly grated

- 1 teaspoon curry powder

- ½ teaspoon ground coriander

- ½ zucchini, diced

- 1 can crushed tomatoes

Directions:

1. Place a nonstick frying pan over medium flame and heat through. Once hot, add the oil and swirl to coat.

2. Add the onion and sauté until translucent. Add the garlic and ginger and sauté until fragrant. Stir in the curry powder and coriander and sauté until fragrant.

3. Add the zucchini and tomatoes, then let simmer for about 8 minutes or until zucchini is crisp tender. Serve right away.

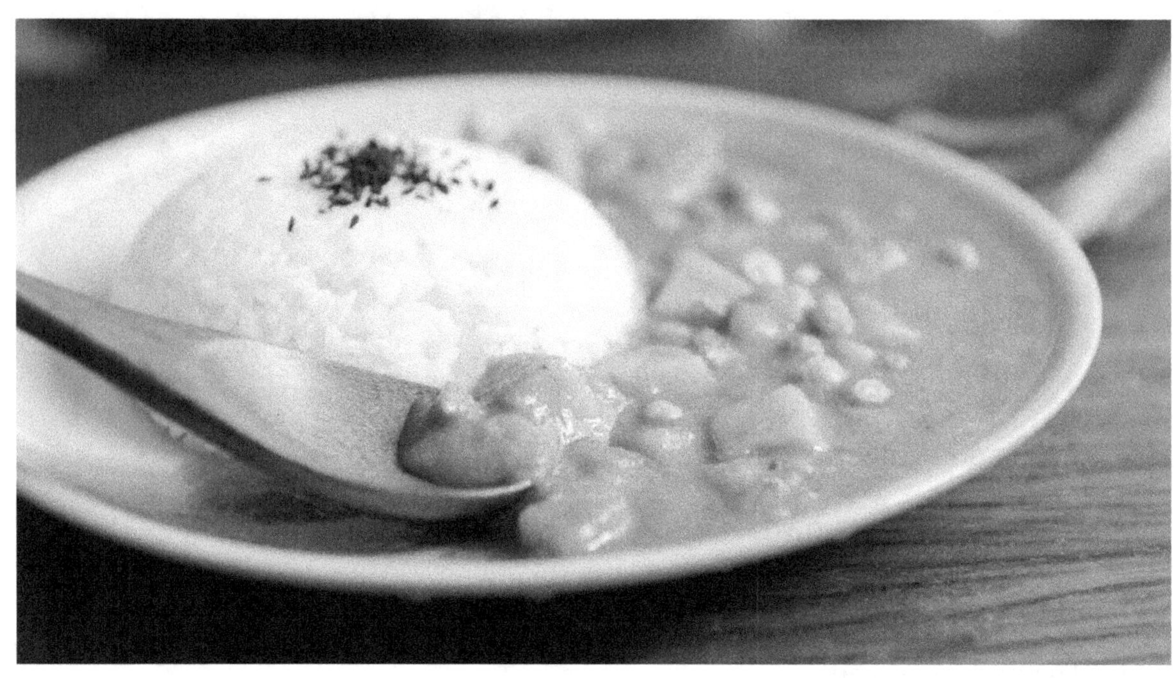

White Chili Bean

Ingredients:

- 4 cups freshly boiled water

- 2 dried white beans, drained

- 3 garlic, minced

- 1 white onion, minced

- 1 banana chili, minced

- 1 can canned, diced tomatoes

- 1½ tablespoon chili powder

- 1½ tablespoons cumin powder

- ½ teaspoon liquid smoke hickory seasoning

- Pinch of kosher salt

Directions:

1. Except for canned tomatoes and tomato paste, pour remaining ingredients into slow cooker set at medium heat. Stir; secure lid. Cook for 6 hours, or until beans are fork tender. Turn off heat.

2. Stir in remaining ingredients. Let dish rest for 15 minutes, covered. Ladle recommended serving into bowls. Serve.

Hearty Rice and Peas

Ingredients:

- 2 cups white long-grained Japanese sticky rice, drained

- 1 cup frozen peas, thawed

- 1 can whole button mushrooms, quartered

- 2 tablespoons trail mix

- ⅛ teaspoon Spanish paprika powder

- Pinch of kosher salt

- Pinch of black pepper

- vegetable stock

Directions:

1. Except for vegetable stock, pour ingredients into rice cooker. Pour stock until liquid reaches 4-cup line of pot. Stir; secure lid. Press cook; wait for machine to automatically shift to warm. Turn off heat.
2. Ladle recommended serving portions into bowls. Serve warm.

Curried Rice

Ingredients:

- 2 cups brown rice, rinsed

- 1 can coconut cream

- 1 cauliflower, sliced into bite-sized florets

- 1 carrot, diced

- 1 garlic clove, minced

- 1 shallot, minced

- 1 tablespoon curry powder

- Pinch of kosher salt

- vegetable stock

Directions:

1. Pour ingredients into rice cooker. Pour stock until liquid reaches 4-cup line of pot. Stir; secure lid. Press cook; wait for machine to automatically shift to warm. Turn off heat.

2. Ladle recommended serving portions into bowls. Serve.

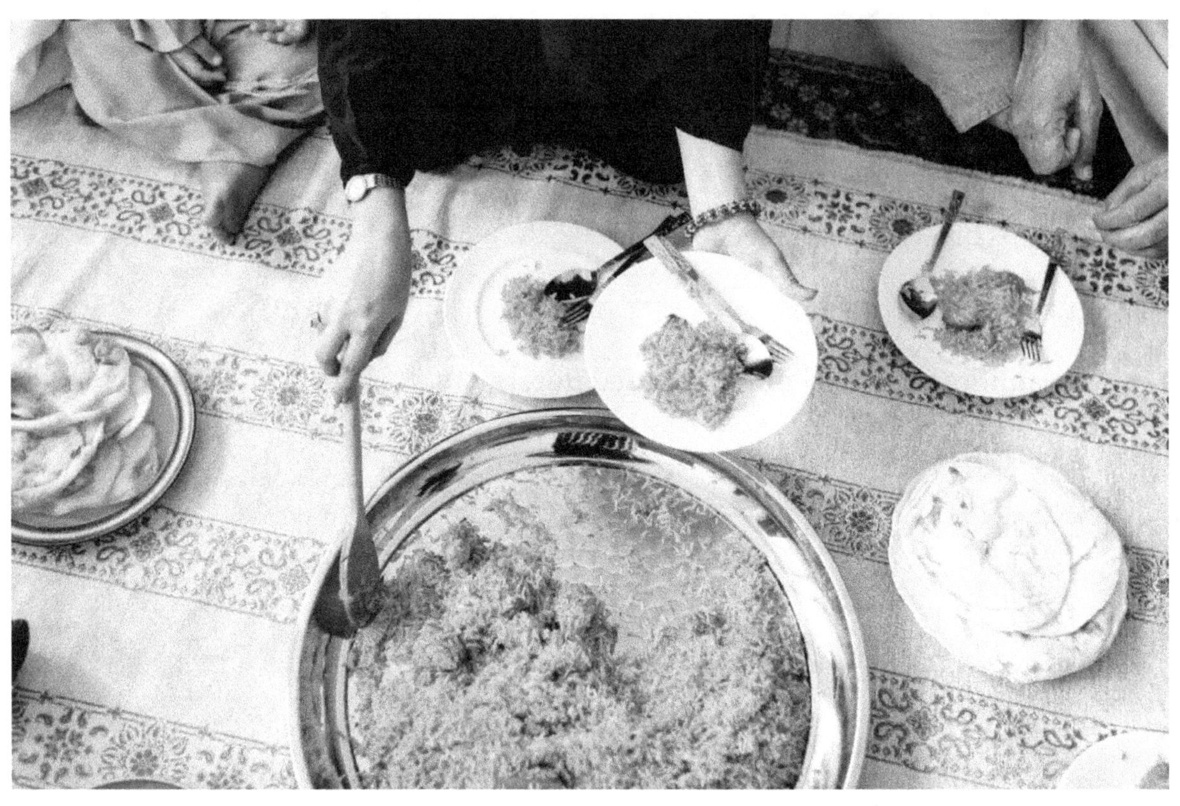

Zucchini Red Sauce

Ingredients:

- 2 tablespoon olive oil, add more if needed
- ¼ tablespoon oregano powder
- 2 zucchinis, diced
- 2 garlic cloves, minced
- 1 can diced and peeled tomatoes
- ¼ cup frozen whole corn kernels, thawed
- ¼ cup fresh basil leaves, chopped
- Pinch of palm sugar
- Pinch of kosher salt
- Pinch of white pepper

Directions:

1. Pour oil into Dutch oven set over medium heat. Stir-fry aubergine until golden brown on all sides.
2. Add in remaining ingredients; let sauce boil away until liquid is reduced by a quarter, or until thickened to desired consistency.
3. Taste; adjust seasoning, if needed. Turn off heat. Serve on top of boiled/steamed rice, or vegetable noodles with vegan cheese, if desired.

Spinach Curry Sauce

Ingredients:

- 2 cans coconut cream, divided
- 2 cups mushroom stock
- 1-pound frozen spinach leaves, thawed
- 1 tablespoon Thai curry paste
- 1 garlic clove, minced
- 1 green chili, chopped
- 1 shallot, minced
- 1 sweet potato, cubed
- Pinch of kosher salt
- Pinch of white pepper

Directions:

1. Except for 1 can of coconut cream, pour ingredients into Dutch oven set over high heat. Stir. Let sauce boil away until liquid is reduced by half. Pour in remaining can of coconut cream. Turn off heat immediately.

2. Cool completely before processing into blender until smooth. Taste; adjust seasoning, if needed.

3. Serve on top of boiled/steamed rice, or vegetable noodles with vegan cheese, if desired.

Squash Soup with Cashew Cheese

Ingredients:

- 4 cups roasted mushroom stock

- 1 tablespoon olive oil

- 1 garlic clove, minced

- 1 white onion, minced

- 1 butternut squash, cubed

- Pinch of kosher salt

- Pinch of white pepper

For garnish

- ¼ cup cashew cheese

- ¼ cup fresh parsley, minced

Directions:

1. Pour oil into Dutch oven set over medium heat. When oil is hot enough, add in and sauté onion and garlic until limp and aromatic.

2. Except for garnishes, add in remaining ingredients. Stir. Bring soup to a boil. Secure lid. Turn down heat. Simmer for 45 minutes. Turn off heat.

3. Cool slightly before processing into a blender until smooth. Taste; adjust seasoning, if needed.

4. Cool slightly before ladling into bowls. Add equal portions of garnishes on top.

CHAPTER 6

Snacks and Desserts Vegan Keto Recipes

Crispy Kale Leaves

Ingredients:

- 1-pound kale leaves, torn

- olive oil for drizzling

- Pinch of sea salt, add more if needed

Directions:

1. Preheat the oven to 300°F. Line a baking sheet with aluminum foil.

2. Layer kale leaves. Drizzle in olive oil. Bake for 15 minutes or until crisp.

3. Remove from the oven. Cool before serving.

Sweet Avocado Salad

Ingredients:

- 2 ripe avocados, cubed

- ½ cup honey, add more if desired

- 1 can evaporated milk

Directions:

1. Using a large salad bowl, put together avocado, honey, and evaporated milk. Mix well.

2. Place inside the fridge for 1 hour or until ready to eat.

3. To serve: ladle equal amounts into salad bowls.

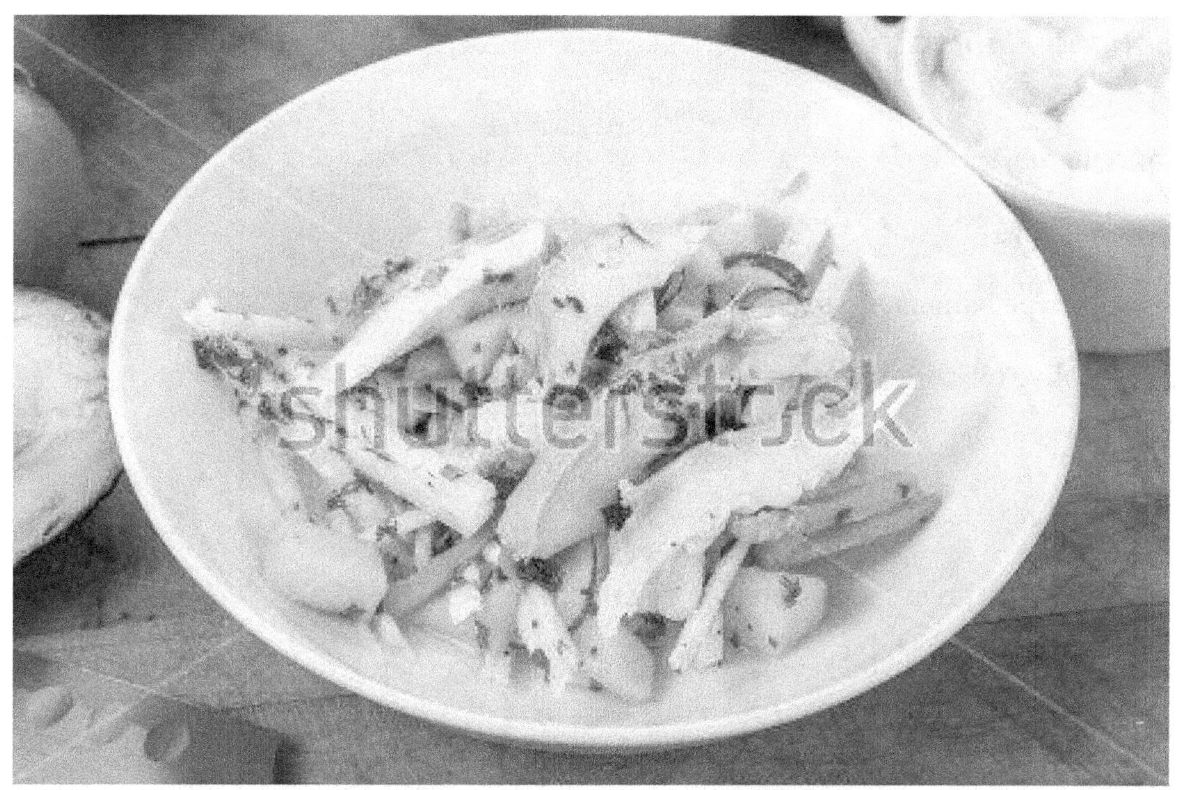

Banana Flapjacks

Ingredients:

- 2 eggs

- 1 ripe banana, mashed

- olive oil, for greasing and frying

Directions:

1. Lightly grease a non-stick frying pan.

2. Meanwhile, whisk mashed banana and together. Continue mixing until a watery and buttery consistency is achieved. Divide batter into equal portions.

3. Pour on a hot pan. You will know that flapjacks are cooked when the edges are golden and set. Cook for a total time of 2 minutes.

4. Stack cooked flapjacks on a plate. Serve immediately.

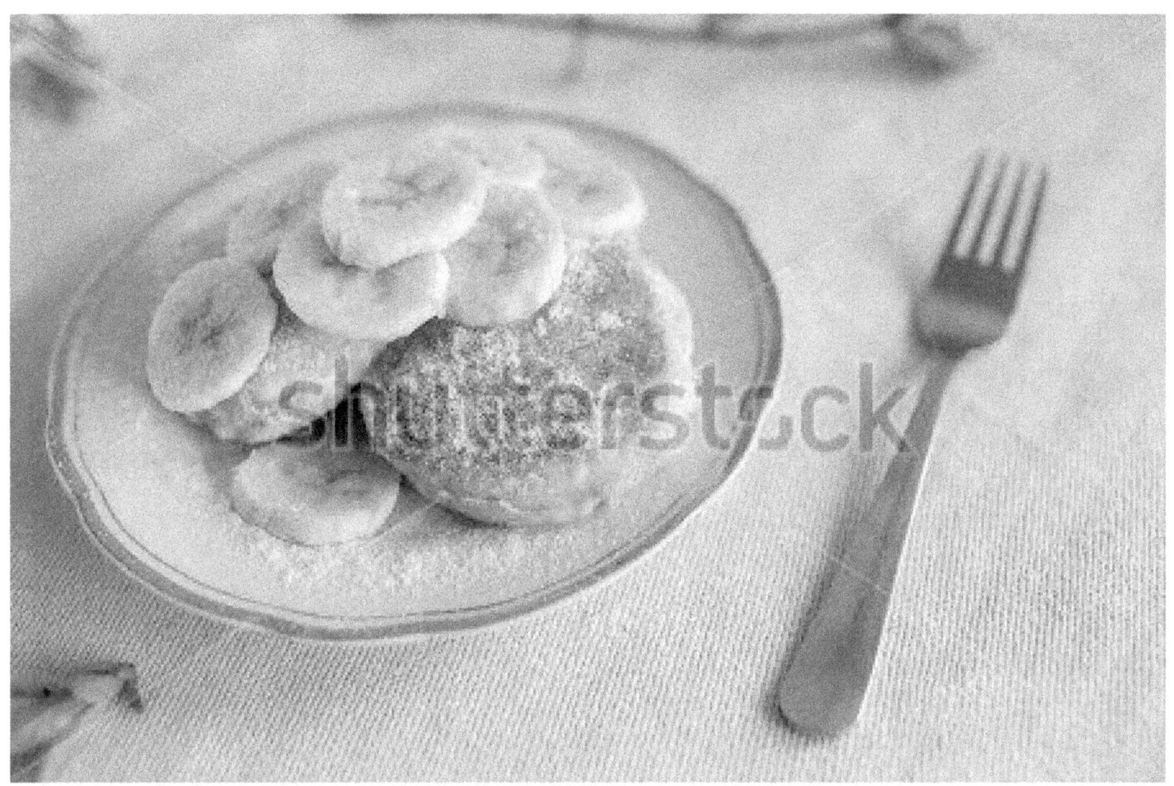

www.shutterstock.com · 409765495

Homemade Pickled Cucumber

Ingredients:

For the pickles:

- 4 garlic cloves, smashed

- 1 tsp. dried dill leaves

- 4 cucumbers, sliced into thick disks

- 1 dried bay leaf

For the pickling brine:

- 1 garlic clove, smashed

- 1 tsp. mustard seeds

- ½ cup white wine vinegar

- 2 tsp. honey

- Pinch of sea salt, add more if needed

Directions:

1. For the pickling brine, put together garlic clove, mustard seeds, white wine vinegar, honey, and salt in a large saucepan. Bring mixture to a boil. Turn off the heat and allow to cool at room temperature.

2. For the pickles, pack garlic cloves, dill leaves, cucumbers, and bay leaf in a mason jar.

3. Pour the prickling brine into the jar. Seal.

4. Let cool completely at room temperature before placing inside the fridge for 2 hours or until needed.

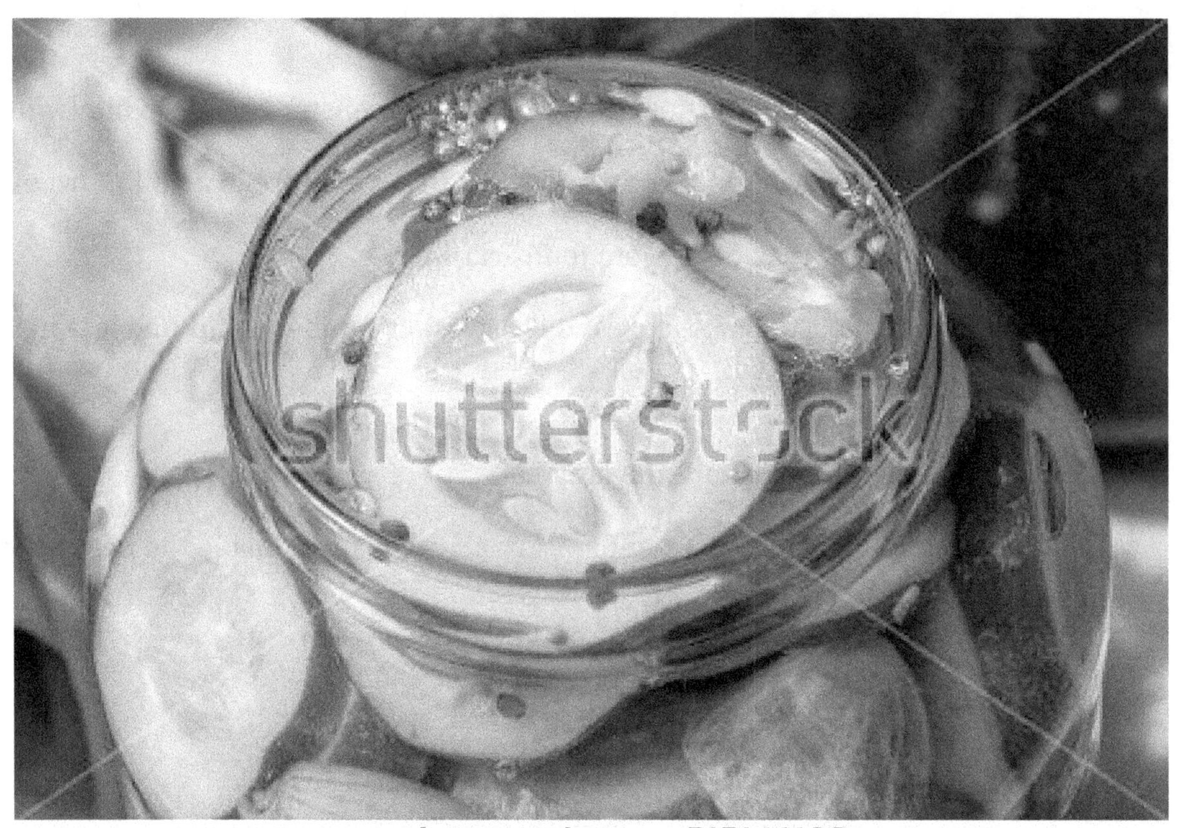

www.shutterstock.com · 517144198

Pickled Vegetables

Ingredients:

For the Vegetables:

- water, for boiling vegetables
- Pinch of sea salt, add more if needed
- 1 cauliflower head, cut into bite-sized florets
- 1 carrot, sliced into thick coins
- 1 broccoli head, cut into bite-sized florets
- 4 onions, leave whole
- 4 garlic cloves, leave whole
- 6 red chili peppers, leave whole
- 1 fennel bulb, thickly sliced
- 1 tsp. fennel seeds
- ½ yellow bell pepper, cut into thick strips
- ½ red bell pepper, cut into thick strips
- ¼ celeriac root, cut into long strips
- 2 Tbsp. capers in brine

For the brine:

- 1 cup white wine vinegar
- Pinch of sea salt, add more if needed
- 1 tsp. black peppercorns
- 1 tsp. Spanish paprika powder
- 1 cup water
- Pinch of white pepper, to taste
- ½ cup honey

For the icy bath:

- 3 cups cold water
- 1 cup, heaping ice cubes

Directions:

1. For the vegetables: fill a Dutch oven with ¾ full of water. Bring water to a boil. Sprinkle salt.

2. Add in cauliflower florets. Cook for 6 minutes or until the veggie turns a shade darker.

3. Remove florets from the boiling water and dunk into an icy bath.

4. Do the same for the broccoli and the carrots.

5. For the brine, combine white wine vinegar, salt, peppercorns, paprika powder, water, and pepper. Bring mixture to a boil. Reduce the heat and allow to simmer until the liquid is reduced by a quarter. Stir in honey. Allow to cool completely at room temperature.

6. For the pickles, drain cooked vegetables from the icy bath. Transfer to a big bowl. Add in onion, garlic, red chili peppers, fennel bulb, fennel seeds, yellow and red bell peppers, celiac root, and capers in brine. Toss mixture until well combined.

7. Pour brine into the veggie bowl. Stir well. Cover with saran wrap. Place inside the fridge for 2 hours before bottling.

8. Pour an equal amount of pickles and brine into jars. Seal. Use as needed.

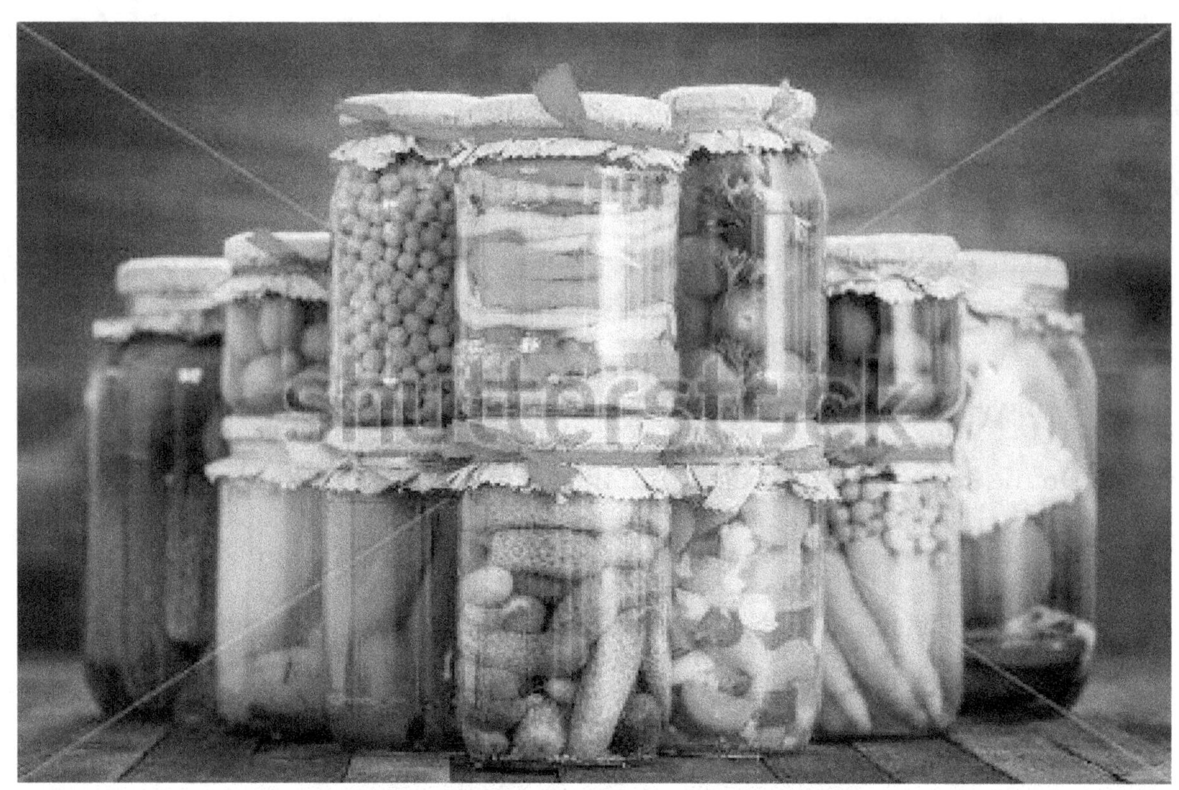

Homemade Parsley and Garlic Butter

Ingredients:

- 4 garlic cloves, grated

- 1 tsp. heaping parsley, minced

- 1 cup butter

Directions:

1. Put together garlic, parsley, and butter in a medium-sized mixing bowl.

2. Place mixture in a non-reactive container with a lid.

3. Chill for 30 minutes to 1 hour. Use as needed.

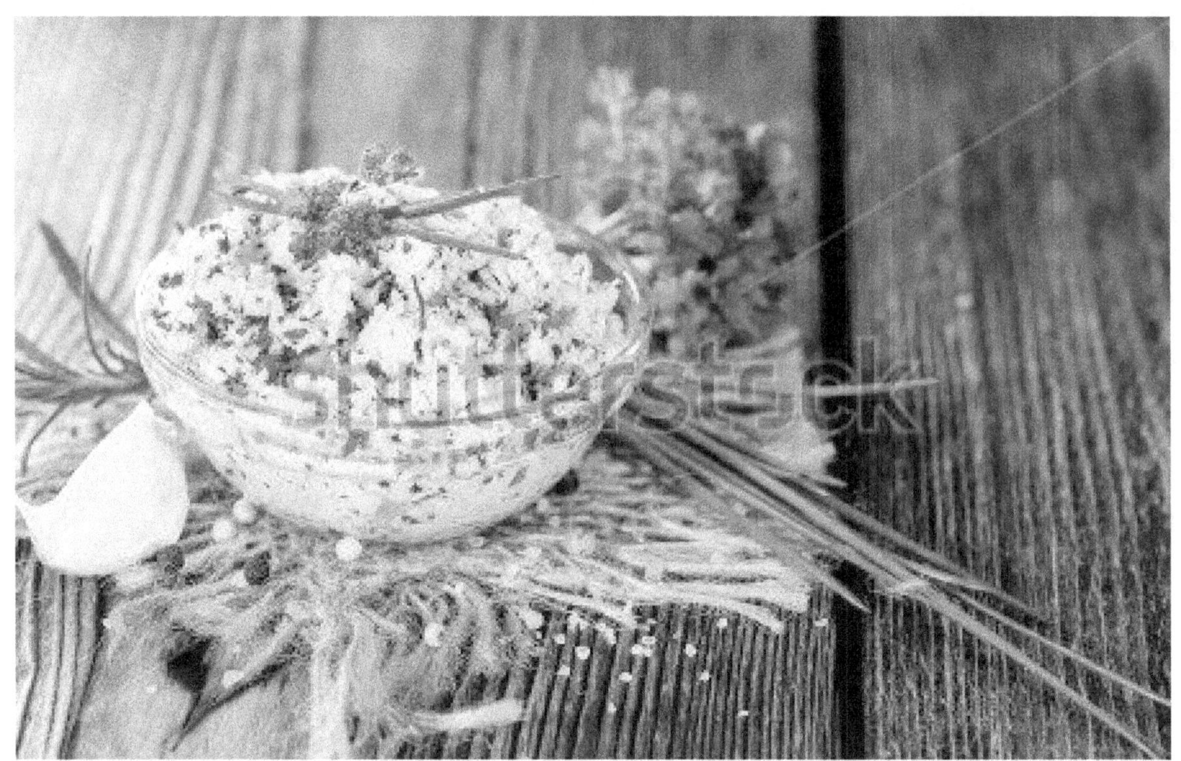

shutterstock
www.shutterstock.com · 241856653

Homemade Rosemary and Cream Cheese Butter

Ingredients:

- 1 garlic clove, grated

- 1 tsp., heaping rosemary, minced

- 1 cup butter, preferably salted

- 1 tsp., heaping cream cheese

- 1 tsp. lime juice, freshly-squeezed

Directions:

1. Put together garlic, rosemary, butter, cream cheese, and leim juice in a medium-sized mixing bowl.

2. Place mixture in a non-reactive container with a lid.

3. Chill for 30 minutes to 1 hour. Use as needed.

Homemade Basil, Cashew, and Garlic Butter

Ingredients:

- 1 garlic clove, grated

- 1 fresh basil, minced

- 1 cup butter, preferably salted

- 1 tsp., heaping cashew nuts, roasted, chopped

- Pinch of white pepper, to taste

Directions:

1. Put together garlic, basil, butter, cashew nuts, and white pepper in a medium-sized mixing bowl.

2. Place mixture in a non-reactive container with a lid.

3. Chill for 30 minutes to 1 hour. Use as needed.

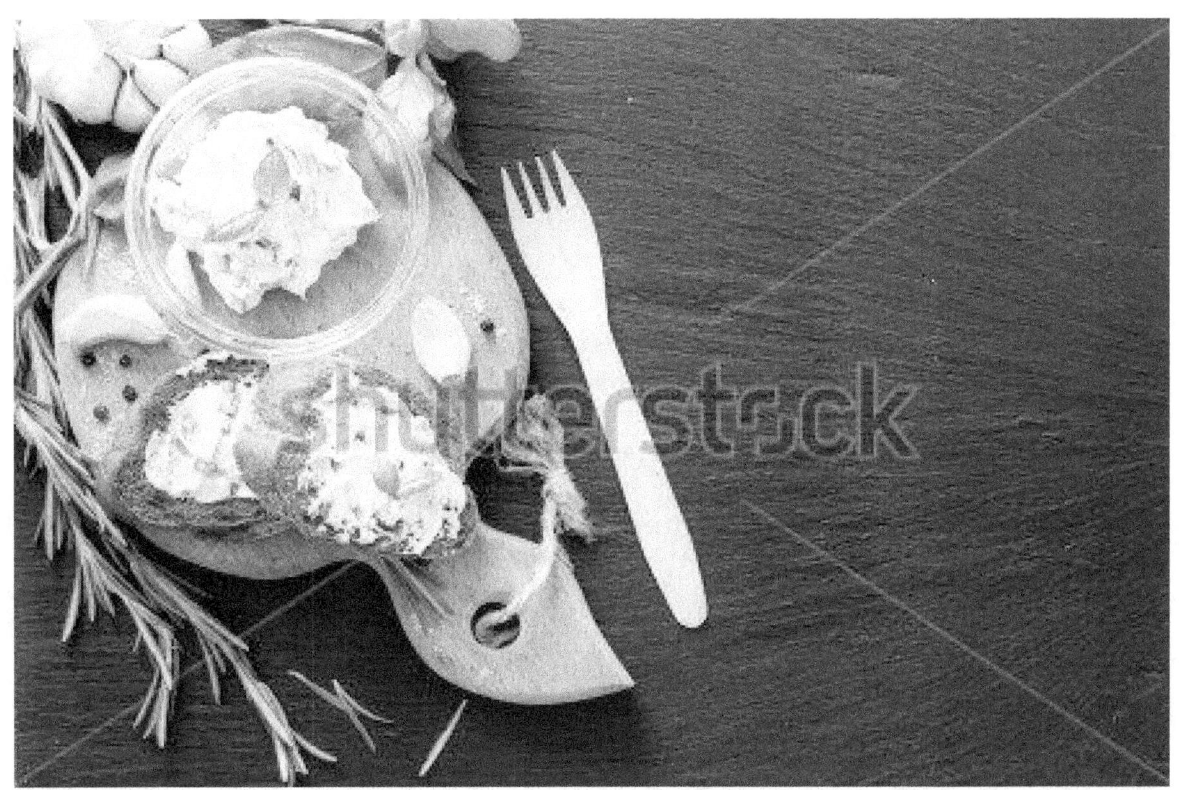
www.shutterstock.com · 291284417

Sundried Tomato Butter

Ingredients:

- 1 Tbsp. sundried tomatoes, minced

- ⅛ cup fresh basil leaves, minced

- 1 cup butter

- Pinch of sea salt, add more if needed

- Pinch of white pepper, to taste

Directions:

1. Put together sundried tomatoes, basil leaves, butter, salt, and pepper in a medium-sized mixing bowl.

2. Place mixture in a non-reactive container with a lid.

3. Chill for 30 minutes to 1 hour. Use as needed.

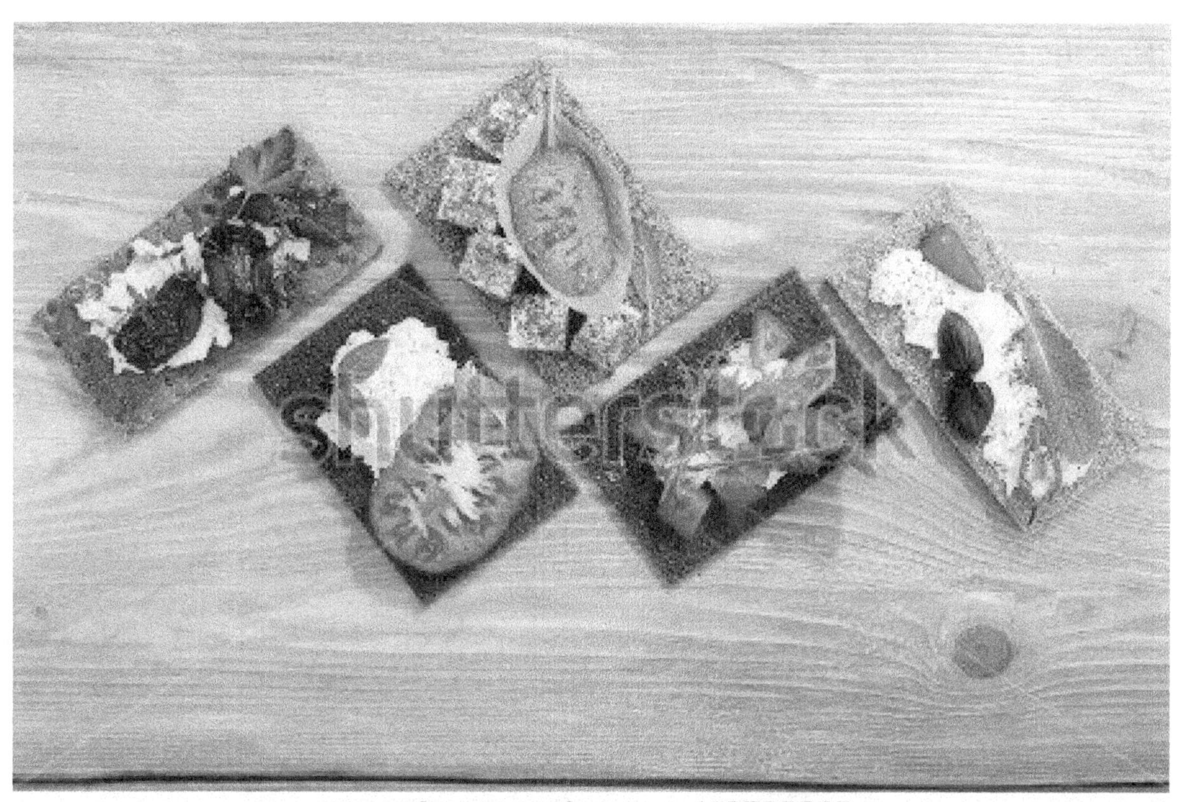

Bruschetta with Parmesan and Basil-Tomato Spread

Ingredients:

- 2 slices grain-free almond-coconut bread, toasted on both sides
- 2 garlic cloves, peeled
- extra virgin olive oil, for drizzling
- balsamic vinegar, for drizzling
- Parmesan cheese shavings

Tomato spread

- 1 tomato, minced
- 2 fresh basil leaves, minced
- 1 tsp. fresh chives, for garnish
- Pinch of sea salt

Directions:

1. To make tomato spread: lightly salt tomatoes; place in strainer to drain for at least 5 minutes prior to use. Combine with basil leaves and chives.
2. Rub garlic cloves on toasted bread slices until these become nubs; discard nubs. Drizzle small amount of balsamic vinegar on bread slices, and then top off with tomato spread.
3. Add desired amount of Parmesan cheese shavings on each slice.
4. Warm bread slices in oven toaster on highest heat setting for 3 to 5 minutes. Transfer bruschetta to a plate. Drizzle in olive oil just before serving.

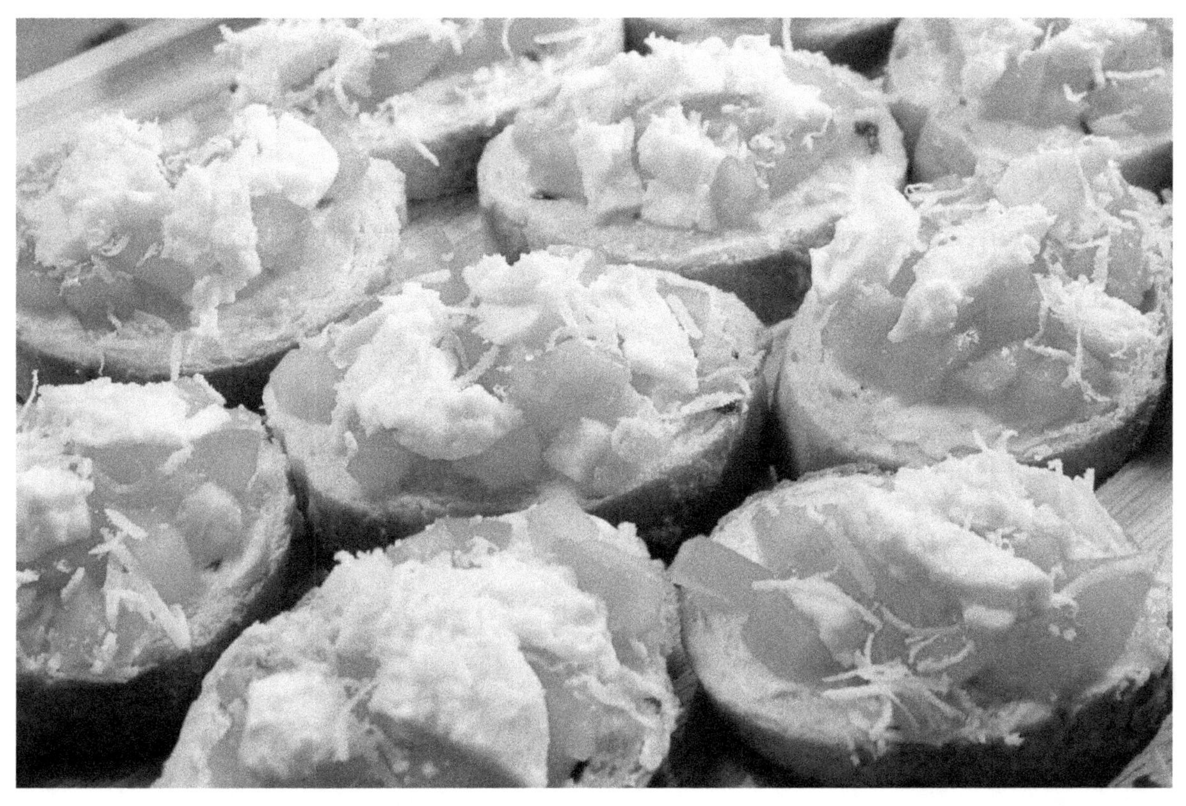

Coco Peanut Truffles

Ingredients:

- 1 ½ cups dates, pitted, chopped, soaked in water for 10 minutes

- 1 ½ cups walnuts

- 1/3 cup cacao powder

- 1/3 cup coconut, shredded

- 1 ½ Tbsp. peanut butter

Directions:

1. Drain the soaked dates, then place in a food processor. Add the peanut butter, cacao powder, and nuts. Blend until pasty.

2. Add the shredded coconut and blend again until combined.

3. Roll the batter into one-inch balls and arrange on a tray. Place in the refrigerator and chill until firm. Serve chilled.

Vegan Brownies

Ingredients:

- ¾ cup all-purpose flour
- ½ Tbsp. baking powder
- ¼ cup vegan margarine
- 5 oz pureed prune
- 1 cup light brown sugar
- 3 oz chocolate, unsweetened
- 1 tsp pure vanilla extract

Directions:

1. Preheat the oven to 350 degrees F. Line a small baking pan with aluminum foil and set aside.
2. Place the margarine and chocolate in a microwaveable bowl and microwave over medium heat until completely melted.
3. Carefully remove the mixture from the microwave and stir in the pureed prune and light brown sugar.
4. In a bowl, combine the baking powder and flour. Fold in the chocolate mixture, then stir in the vanilla. Mix everything well until thoroughly incorporated.
5. Pour the batter in the prepared baking pan, packing tightly using a rubber spatula. Bake for 12 to 15 minutes, or until the brownies are firm.
6. Set on a cooling rack and allow to cool. Slice into even squares and serve, or store in an airtight container.

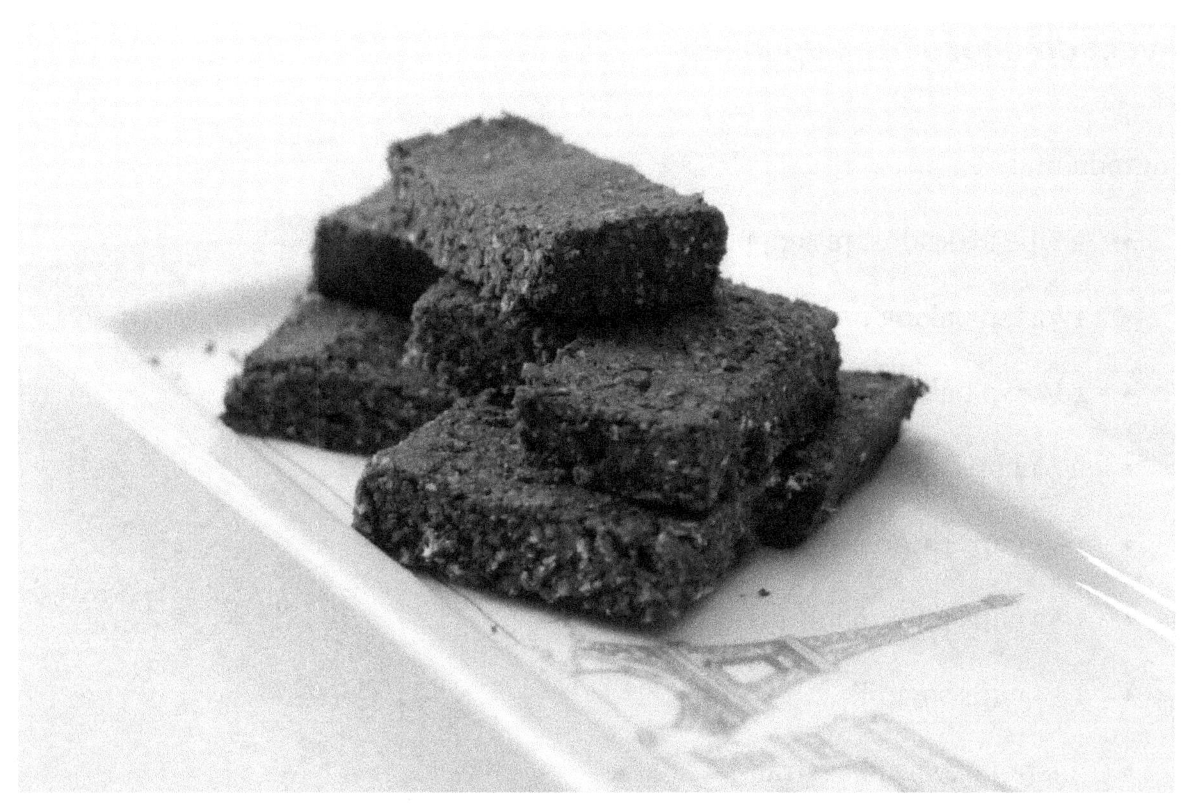

Avocado Chocolate Cupcakes

Ingredients:

- 2 ripe avocados, pitted, peeled
- 1 ½ tsp baking powder
- 1 ¼ tsp baking soda
- 2 ¼ cups all-purpose flour
- 1 ¼ cups cacao powder
- 1 ½ cups pure maple syrup
- 1 ¼ cups soymilk
- 3 tsp pure vanilla extract
- 1 ¼ tsp sea salt
- 3 tbsp. olive oil

For the Chocolate Cream:

- 4.5 oz soft silken tofu, drained
- 6 oz cacao nibs, melted
- ¾ tsp pure vanilla extract
- 4 ½ Tbsp. pure maple syrup
- 1/6 tsp sea salt

Directions:

1. Set the oven to 350 degrees F. line 16 cupcake tins with paper liners and set aside.

2. Combine the cacao powder, flour, baking soda, baking powder, and salt in a bowl.

3. Mash the avocado until smooth, then stir in the vanilla extract, oil, and maple syrup. Combine the flour and avocado mixture.

4. Divide the batter among the cupcake tins, then bake for 25 minutes. Insert a toothpick in the center of a cupcake; if it comes out clean, the cupcakes are done.

5. Set on a cooling rack and allow to cool slightly before serving.

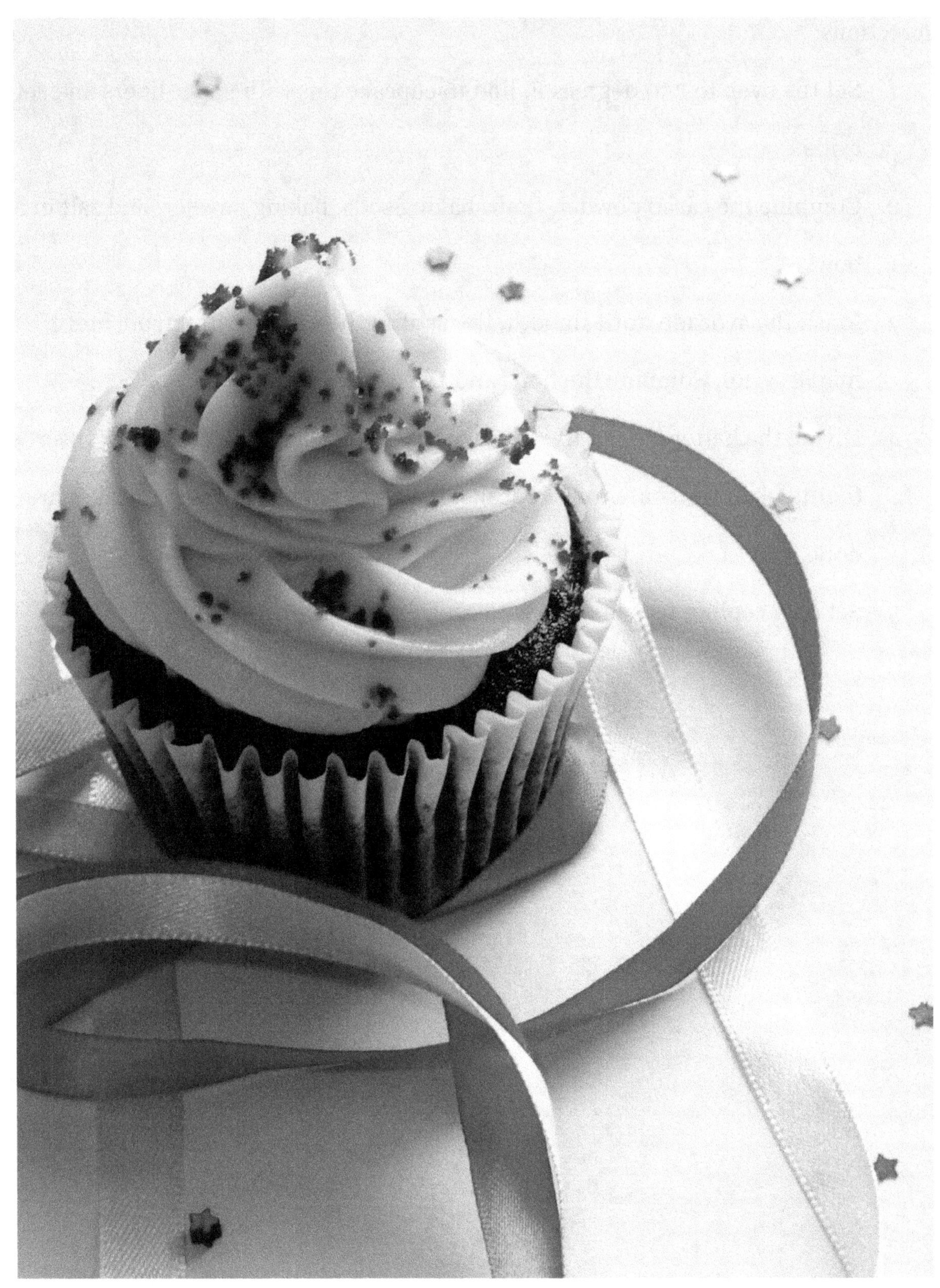

Slow Cooked Cinnamon Apples

Ingredients:

- 4 baking apples, cored, halved

- 1 ½ vanilla beans

- 1 ½ cinnamon sticks

- 3 inches fresh ginger, peeled

- ¾ cups water

Directions:

1. Arrange the apples in a large slow cooker. Pour in the water and spices.

2. Cover and cook for 8 hours on low, or until the apples are fork tender.

3. Transfer the apples onto a platter and serve warm.

Crispy Kale Chips

Ingredients:

- 1 lb. kale leaves, torn

- Pinch of sea salt, to taste coconut oil, melted, for drizzling

-

Directions:

1. Preheat oven to 300°F/150°C for at least 10 minutes. Line 2 baking sheets with parchment paper.

2. Toss kale leaves and coconut oil into a bowl to combine; spread leaves as flat as possible on baking sheets. Season lightly with salt; drizzle in more oil.

3. Bake for 15 to 20 minutes or until kale turns a shade darker; remove from oven. Cool slightly before serving.

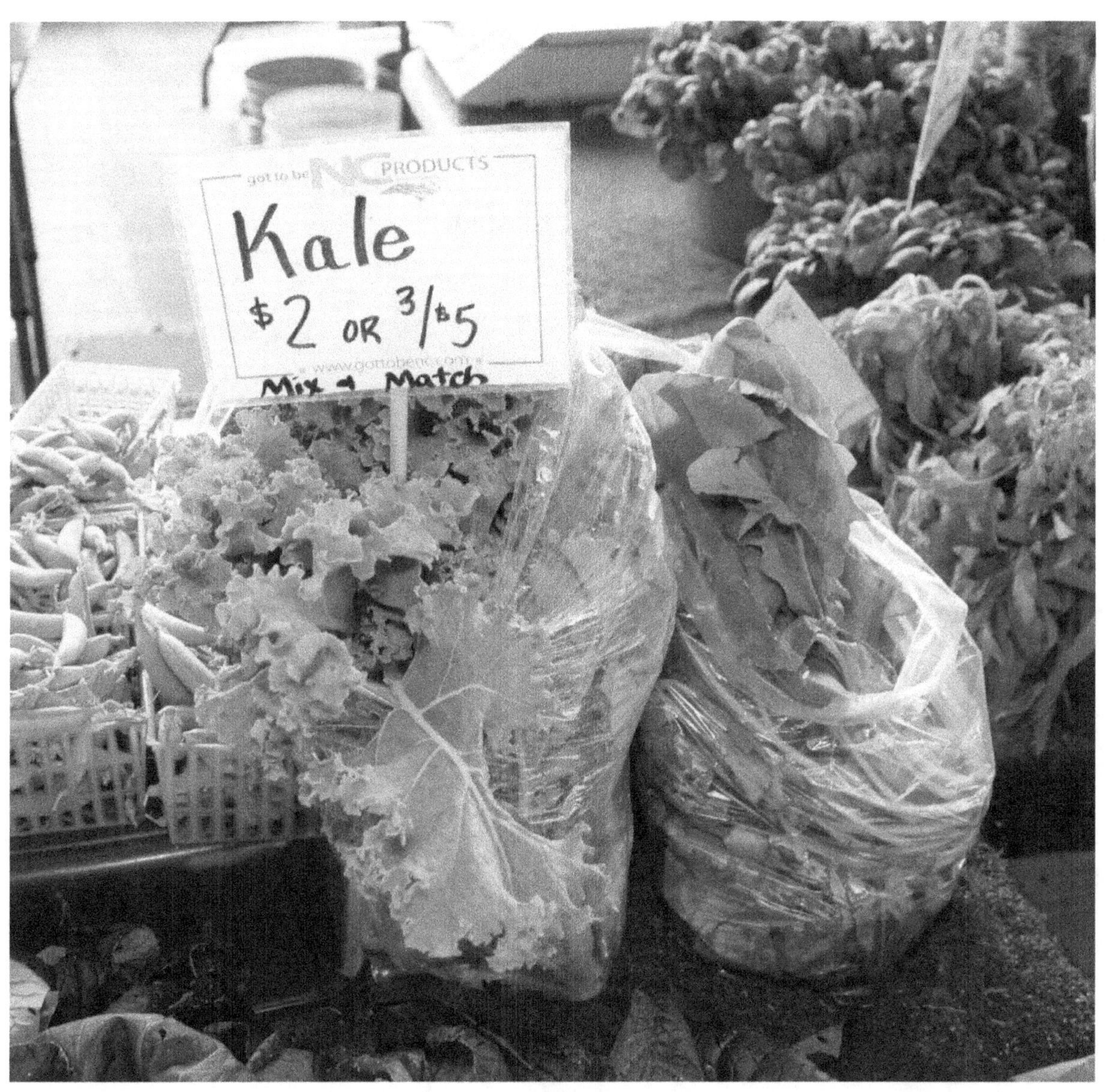

got to be NC PRODUCTS
Kale
$2 OR 3/$5
www.gottobenc.com
Mix + Match

Sun-Dried Tomatoes and Basil Spread

Ingredients:

- 2 slices thick ketogenic safe bread, toasted
- 2 garlic cloves, peeled
- ⅛ teaspoon avocado oil

Toppings

- 1 fresh tomato, diced
- 4 fresh basil leaves, julienned
- 2 sun-dried tomatoes in oil, julienned
- Pinch of sea salt
- Pinch of white pepper

Directions:

1. Preheat oven toaster. Rub garlic cloves on both sides of toasted bread. Top slices with equal amounts of basil, fresh tomatoes, and sun-dried tomatoes.
2. Place bread into oven toaster to warm through. Remove from heat.
3. Season lightly with salt and pepper; drizzle in avocado oil just before serving.

CHAPTER 7

30 Days Meal Plan

Day 1

Breakfast - Chia Blueberry Pudding

Lunch - Brussels Sprouts with Lime Dip

Dinner – Chili and Bean Rice

Snack – Homemade Pickled Cucumber

Day 2

Breakfast - Creamy Broccoli Soup

Lunch - Green Beans and Walnuts

Dinner - Broccoli and Cauliflower Stir-Fry

Snack – Banana Flapjacks

Day 3

Breakfast - Plantain Flapjacks

Lunch - Savory Roasted Cabbage

Dinner - Bean Casserole

Snack – Crispy Kale Leaves

Day 4

Breakfast - Veggie Tofu Scramble

Lunch - Tofu Tacos

Dinner - Breaded Baby Carrots

Snack – Pickled Vegetables

Day 5

Breakfast - Cardamom Bread

Lunch - Tofu Tacos

Dinner - Courgette Pasta with Mixed Greens and Fruits Salad

Snack – Sweet Avocado Salad

Day 6

Breakfast - Scrambled Eggless Eggs

Lunch - Lasagna Eggplant

Dinner - Chop Suey with Straw Mushrooms

Snack – Homemade Parsley and Garlic Butter

Day 7

Breakfast - Cardamom Bread

Lunch - Veggie Salad in Soy Vinaigrette

Dinner - Baked Onion Rings

Snack - Homemade Basil, Cashew, and Garlic Butter

Day 8

Breakfast - Cranberry and Blueberry Pancakes

Lunch - Bean Burrito

Dinner - Spicy Stuffed Bell Peppers

Snack – Sundried Tomato Butter

Day 9

Breakfast - Raisin Rice Pudding

Lunch - Green Salad with Basil Dressing

Dinner - Cauliflower Pop

Snack – Homemade Rosemary and Cream Cheese Butter

Day 10

Breakfast - Cardamom Pancakes with Chocolate Buttons

Lunch - Veggie Pitas

Dinner - Spiced Cherry Tomatoes and Cucumber Salad

Snack – Bruschetta with Parmesan and Basil-Tomato Spread

Day 11

Breakfast - Morning French Toast

Lunch - Basil Bruschetta with Cashew Cheese

Dinner - Spicy Tofu Paella

Snack – Coco Peanut Truffles

Day 12

Breakfast - Cardamom Pancakes with Chocolate Buttons

Lunch - Squadles (Squash Noodles)

Dinner - Spicy Stuffed Bell Peppers

Snack – Bruschetta with Parmesan and Basil-Tomato Spread

Day 13

Breakfast - Fruit-Filled Muffins

Lunch - Smooth and Spicy Veggie Soup

Dinner - Broccoli and Cauliflower Stir-Fry

Snack – Avocado Chocolate Cupcakes

Day 14

Breakfast - Almond Porridge with Fresh Fruits

Lunch - Veggie Pitas

Dinner - Breaded Artichoke Hearts

Snack – Vegan Brownies

Day 15

Breakfast - Pumpkin and Chocolate Pancakes

Lunch - Boodles (Broccoli Stem Noodles)

Dinner - Zucchini and Tomato Curry

Snack – Crispy Kale Chips

Day 16

Breakfast - Morning French Toast

Lunch - Pumpkin Stew

Dinner - Lentil with Butternut Squash Soup

Snack – Slow Cooked Cinnamon Apples

Day 17

Breakfast - Raisin Rice Pudding

Lunch - Green Beans and Walnuts

Dinner - Three Mushroom Quinoa Congee

Snack – Homemade Rosemary and Cream Cheese Butter

Day 18

Breakfast - Pumpkin and Chocolate Pancakes

Lunch - Veggie Pitas

Dinner - Celery and Kale Tiger Salad

Snack – Banana Flapjacks

Day 19

Breakfast - Cardamom Pancakes with Chocolate Buttons

Lunch - Squadles (Squash Noodles)

Dinner - Squash Soup with Cashew Cheese

Snack – Homemade Pickled Cucumber

Day 20

Breakfast - Veggie Tofu Scramble

Lunch - Tofu Tacos

Dinner - Zucchini and Tomato Curry

Snack – Crispy Kale Leaves

Day 21

Breakfast - Scrambled Eggless Eggs

Lunch - Basil Bruschetta with Cashew Cheese

Dinner - Hearty Rice and Peas

Snack – Sweet Avocado Salad

Day 22

Breakfast - Plantain Flapjacks

Lunch - Lasagna Eggplant

Dinner - White Chili Bean

Snack – Sun-Dried Tomatoes and Basil Spread

Day 23

Breakfast - Pumpkin and Chocolate Pancakes

Lunch - Bean Burrito

Dinner - Chop Suey with Straw Mushrooms

Snack – Coco Peanut Truffles

Day 24

Breakfast - Cardamom Pancakes with Chocolate Buttons

Lunch - Green Beans and Walnuts

Dinner - Curried Rice

Snack – Vegan Brownies

Day 25

Breakfast - Veggie Tofu Scramble

Lunch - Tofu Tacos

Dinner - Breaded Baby Carrots

Snack – Bruschetta with Parmesan and Basil-Tomato Spread

Day 26

Breakfast - Cardamom Pancakes with Chocolate Buttons

Lunch - Veggie Pitas

Dinner - Zucchini Red Sauce

Snack – Crispy Kale Leaves

Day 27

Breakfast - Fruit-Filled Muffins

Lunch - Bean Burrito

Dinner - Squash Soup with Cashew Cheese

Snack – Homemade Parsley and Garlic Butter

Day 28

Breakfast - Plantain Flapjacks

Lunch - Green Beans and Walnuts

Dinner - Spicy Stuffed Bell Peppers

Snack – Homemade Pickled Cucumber

Day 29

Breakfast - Scrambled Eggless Eggs

Lunch - Squadles (Squash Noodles)

Dinner - Chop Suey with Straw Mushrooms

Snack – Slow Cooked Cinnamon Apples

Day 30

Breakfast - Fruit-Filled Muffins

Lunch - Basil Bruschetta with Cashew Cheese

Dinner - Zucchini and Tomato Curry

Snack - Vegan Brownies

Conclusion

I hope the recipes you found in this cookbook have given you inspiration and ideas for your next meal or those that you can cook for family and friends who would also want to try the Vegan-Keto diet.

Hopefully this cookbook has inspired you to start the vegan and keto diet and turn these recipes as often as you can to create meal plans that will keep you from running out of ideas on what to have for breakfast, lunch, dinner, and snacks.

Finally, serve your family and friends with your best version of these recipes and experience firsthand that you do not have to contribute to animal cruelty to enjoy a delicious meal.

BONUS CONTENT

MEAL PREP CHAPTER 2

On Mindful Eating and Curbing Hunger

Switching to a healthier lifestyle, especially after you've been used to doing things a particular way for so long will take some adjustment. There will be challenges and you might find yourself falling behind at certain points—understand that this is totally fine. What matters is that you get back on track, exert a bit more effort, and make some necessary changes that will support the kind of life you want to have.

When it comes to eating healthier, it's more than just selecting the right food and doing portion control. Your overall mental approach matters just as much and being mindful about how you do things can really help make things easier. With that said, here are a few Do's and Don'ts to keep in mind.

The Do's

1.	Do start with your shopping list.

Always take your time and make sure you feel focused when writing your list. Mindfulness is key when it comes to creating the right grocery list that will benefit your goals. Think about how you've been feeling lately—what does your body require at the moment? With that in mind, start putting together your choices and edit it as you go.

2.	Do savor your meals.

Here's the thing, most people actually rush through their meals because of various reasons. Some may not have a lot of time to spare, whilst there are those who want to use that time for something else "more important". However, it is important to relish your food; take the time to enjoy its flavor, its aroma, and chew properly. Eating mindfully also makes you feel sated for a longer period of time.

3.	Do the "mouth full, hands empty" mantra.

This means that you should set your cutlery down in between mouthfuls of food. Quite similar to the previous tip, this is meant to help slow your eating and enable you to better appreciate your food. Not only that, doing this can actually help increase the response of your gut peptides. You'll feel full for longer and keep you from overeating.

4.	Always wait a minute or two before going back for seconds.

This allows the food you just ate to settle down and give you enough time to think if you really want more. Most people have a tendency to immediately go for seconds right after eating, especially if the food is something they really like. However, this often leads to them feeling too full and bloated. So, take your time after finishing your plate. Have some water or a sip of tea, then decide if you really need to refill your plate.

5.	Do keep your bigger serving bowls of food off the table and out of sight.

This is to serve the previous step's purpose. If you cannot immediately see or reach the food, you won't be able to refill your plate quickly. It also keeps you from craving more just because you keep seeing food. As you may or may not know, just the mere visual of delicious food can make us overeat. If we can see it and smell even while eating, we're bound to grab more servings.

The Don'ts

6.   Don't eat while you're distracted by something.

A lot of us fall into the trap of multi-tasking; in this case, eating whilst doing something else. Maybe you do it while you're watching TV, while you're working, or while you're moving from one place to the next. Sure, it feels good to be accomplishing a lot of things at the same time, but did you know that this can be detrimental to your fitness goals? By doing this, you're likelier to overeat or end up snacking again later. This is because your brain isn't fully processing the fact that you're eating.

So next time, give yourself an hour or 30 minutes to eat your meals.

7.   Don't drink too much alcohol before you begin eating.

Aside from its calorie content, research has shown that people who drink more before eating are actually more prone to cheating on their diets. Alcohol is also known to stimulate are appetites, making it harder for us to say no to food we cannot have.

8.   Don't eat when you're feeling stressed.

A lot of us have a tendency to "eat our feelings" as a means of relieving stress or any emotional distress we may be experiencing. Whilst this does seem to work, it can also cause us to overeat and feel guilty later on. Instead of turning to food during stressful moments, try mindfulness meditation instead. This will help turn our attention away from what we're craving (usually very indulgent food items) and is also a healthier alternative to stress eating.

9.   Don't forego your diet just because you're eating out.

As we've already established, there are ways of still following your diet even when you're out with friends. Remember, people also tend to eat more when they're in social settings or surrounded by friends. Don't stress yourself out when the menu for an event or a restaurant does not fit into your WW freestyle diet. Where you might not be able to be pickier of what you eat, you can always opt for portion sizes.

Eating mindfully is one thing, but the real challenge often happens when you're trying to beat hunger. It can make just about anyone restless and even cranky— everyone's familiar with this. Here are a few do's and don'ts to keep in mind when it comes to curbing your hunger:

The Do's

10.   Do your best to always get enough sleep.

Not getting enough sleep actually affects the balance of your hormones related to the appetite. Research shows that people who have had less than 5 hours of sleep experienced an increase in the ghrelin levels in their body. This is the hormone which actually triggers appetite and decreases leptin levels. Leptin is the hormone that signals our brain when we've had enough food.

11.   Do a bit of cardio after eating.

Doing this has a positive effect on our satiety hormones, helping promote a longer feeling of satiety. Research also proves that doing moderate-intensity exercises can curb feelings of hunger. It is also an effective form of distraction, keeping you from unintentionally eating or snacking.

When you start feeling the need to snack, try going for a walk instead. After you get back from it, you're bound to feel less inclined to grab a bag of chips or snack on your favorite treats. Note that the brain actually enjoys when we form new habits so do try and focus on making healthier ones, instead of trying to break your current bad habits. You'll eventually replace them when the good habits stick.

12.   Do have a hearty breakfast.

Breakfast is important—essential to our day. Having a hearty one provides our body with the ample fuel it needs to give you a head start on the day. People who begin their day with a protein-rich breakfast are less likely to begin craving snacks halfway through their morning. It also keeps you from overeating when lunchtime comes around, effectively preventing body fat gain and enabling you to manage your hunger better.

The Don'ts

13.   Don't eat too many fatty foods.

Having too much dietary fat in your daily meals can actually trigger ghrelin, the hunger hormone. Basically, the fattier the food you eat is, the greater your appetite for it would become. Just think back to all the times you've eaten food like French fries, pizzas, steaks, and so on—it's usually really hard to stop, right? This is why.

Another thing to pay attention to is your low-fat food's total energy content. These types of food is likely to contain great amounts of sugar to compensate for any flavor that's lost due to the low-fat content.

14.   Don't deprive yourself of your favorite foods.

It's totally okay to enjoy the foods you love, but make sure you do so moderately. Doing so actually helps you deal with cravings better and makes you feel less guilty about having them as well. Banning a food only serves to increase your craving for it so don't be afraid to have your favorites whenever you really feel like them.

www.ingramcontent.com/pod-product-compliance
Lightning Source LLC
Chambersburg PA
CBHW081951260726
48657CB00009BA/2559